Bariatric Meal Prep 2023

kristine wilkard

Published by RAJIA AKTER KHATUN, 2022.

BARIATRIC MEAL PREP 2023

First edition. November 8, 2022.

ISBN: 979-8215735589

Written by kristine wilkard.

Table of Contents

Bariatric MEAL PREP 2023
Healthy gastric sleeve & bypass recipes with picture after weigh loss surgery

Kristine Wilkard

Introduction

Gastric sleeve?

The gastric sleeve, also known as laparoscopic sleeve gastrectomy, is a minimally invasive surgical procedure that helps people lose weight by removing around 80% of their stomach.

Bariatric?

The word "bariatric" refers to the treatment, prevention, and causes of obesity when it is applied in a medical environment.

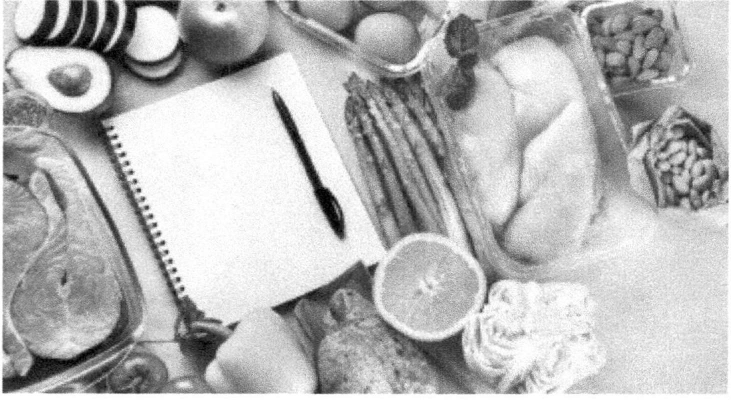

1st stage

CLEAR LIQUIDS DIET

The day following surgery, you'll start a clear liquid diet that will last for about 4-5 days. You should try your hardest to consume 3 ounces of clear liquids every 30 minutes throughout this time. Following your treatment, this could be difficult at first, but with time it will get easier and more comfortable! In order to prevent gas and bloating, avoid using a straw or chewing gum when drinking at this period.

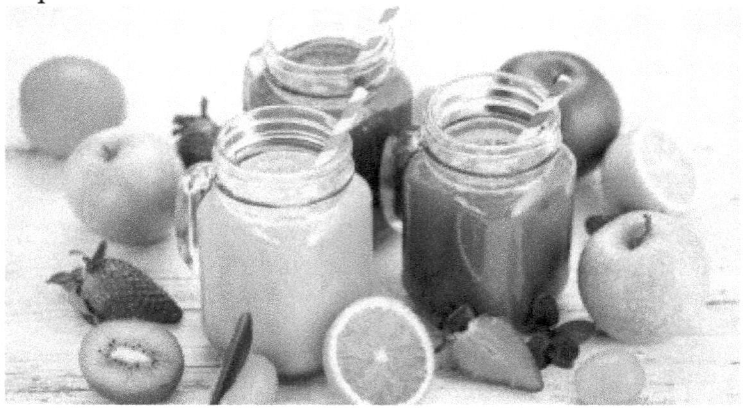

1.protein shake HOMEMADE

prep time 5 min
total time 10 min

Ingredients

- 1 HANDFUL OF SPINACH
- 3...4 STRAWBERRIES
- ½ BANANA
- 1 HANDFUL OF BLUEBERRIES
- WATER
- WHEY PROTEIN POWDER

Instruction

1. Blend all.
2. Serve.

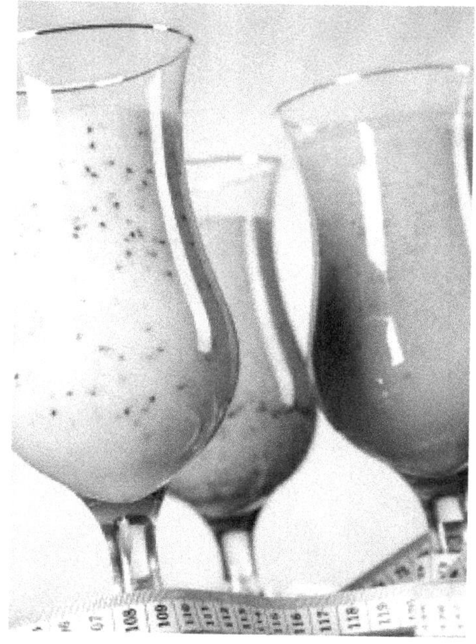

2.Apple juice homemade

Prep time5 mins
Total time10 mins

Ingredients

- Two apple

Instruction

1. Remove apples cover and seeds
2. Cut in pitches
3. Now blend
4. Filter and eat liquid

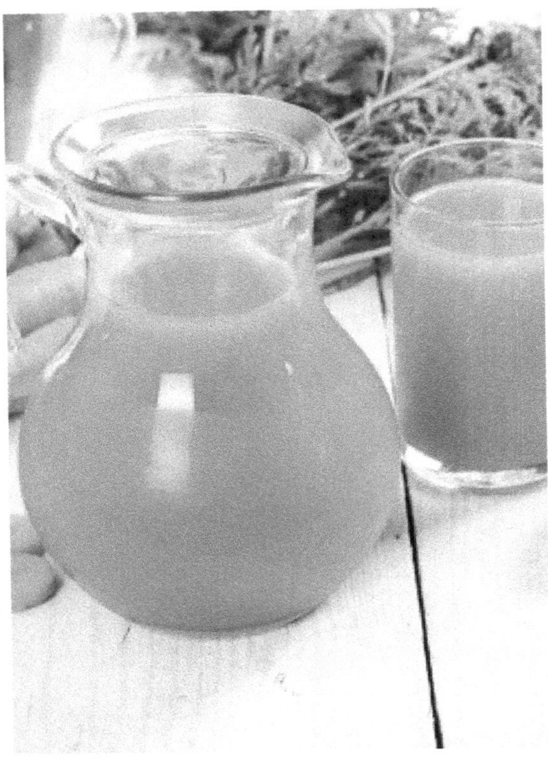

3. Mango Pineapple SMOOthie

Prep time
5 mins

Ingredients

- 1 cup of nonfat Yogurt
- 1/2 cups of frozen pineapple
- 1/2 cups of frozen mango
- 1 cup of ice

Instructions

1. In a blender, add all ingredients perfectly.
2. Mix until smooth.
3. Enjoy immediately.

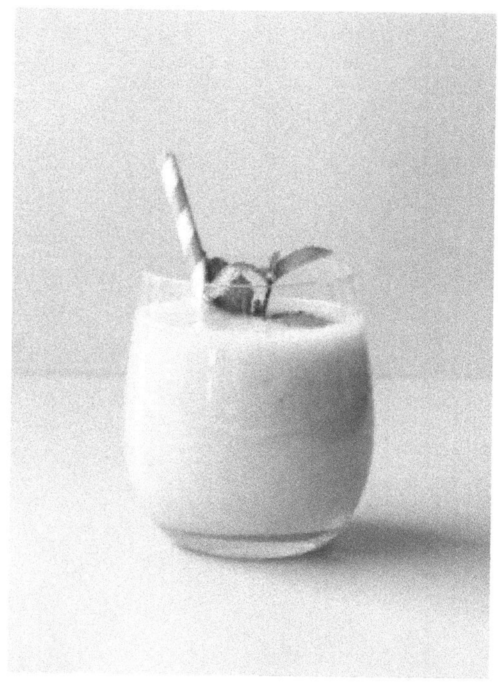

4. Mango Protein Ice Pops HOMEMADE

Ingredients

- 1 cup of whey protein powder,
- 1 cups of yogurt plain, suggest fat-free
- ½ cups of mango fresh or frozen.

Directions:

1. Blend till completely smooth.
2. Pour about 1/2 cup of mixture into each popsicle mold.
3. Freeze for at least one hour or till completely frozen.

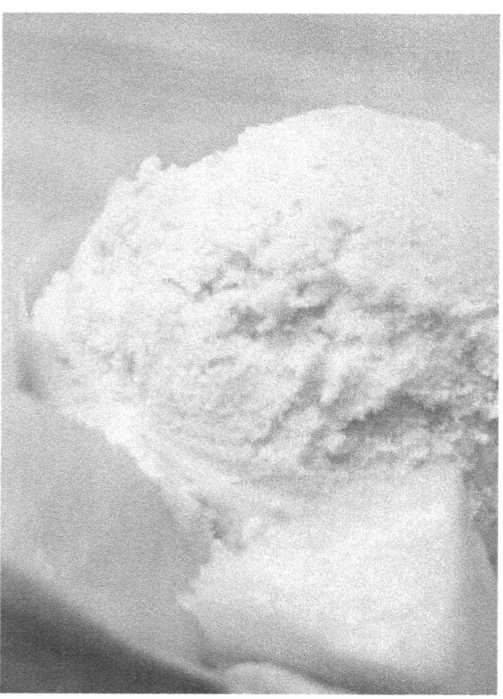

5. Mango SmoOTHIES

Prep Time: 5 Minutes
Total Time: 5 Minutes

INGREDIENTS

- 1 cup peeled and sliced peaches, cold
- Two ice cubes
- 1/2 cup chopped mangoes, cold
- 1/2 of a banana

INSTRUCTIONS

1. In a blender, mix and blend ingredients till smooth.
2. Enjoy cold.

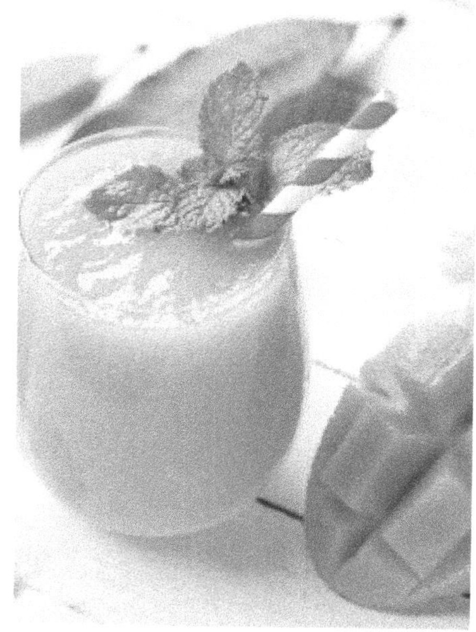

2nd stage

FULL LIQUIDS DIET

You can go to stage two of your diet after around 4-5 days if you can drink 48 ounces of clear liquids per day. Foods that are mushy or have a consistency similar to yogurt are included during this stage, which lasts for about 7 to 10 days. Don't skip any meals and try to eat every 3 to 4 hours. Each of these meals ought to be roughly the size of 12 cups, or two ounces. You should continue to consume at least 48 to 64 ounces of water during this time.

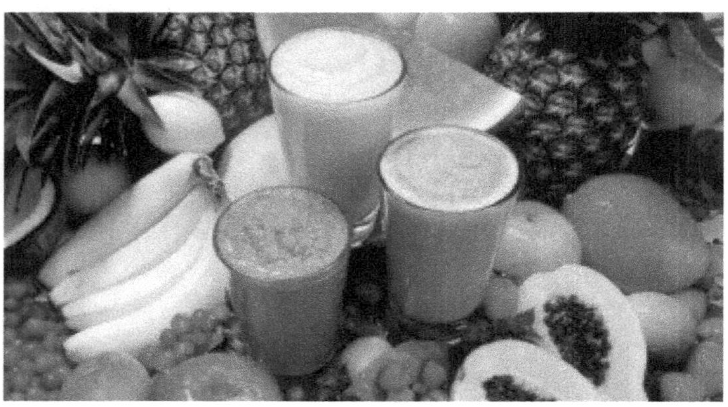

1.Frozen Yogurt

PREP TIME30 mins
FREEZING TIME2 hrs
TOTAL TIME2 hrs 30 mins

INGREDIENTS

- 1 cup of Greek Yogurt, fat sugar-free
- 4 cups of frozen strawberries
- water

INSTRUCTIONS

1. Blend in yogurt, berries, and juice till smooth purée forms.

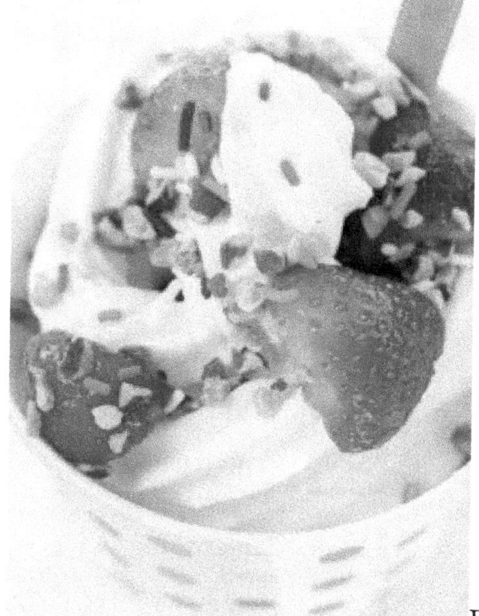

2. Fill a colander with all of the frozen yogurts and place it over a bowl. With a rubber spatula, push all of the yogurts through the sieve, scraping the underside of the sieve to get all of the yogurts into a bowl.
3. Freeze for 2 hours after transferring to serving plates.

2. Key Pie SmoOTHIE

Prep Time5 minutes
Total Time5 minutes

Ingredients

1. One banana sliced and frozen
2. ½ cups of yogurt fat sugar-free
3. water

Instructions

1. Blend all ingredients till smooth, adding ice as required to get the desired consistency.
2. Pour in a smoothie and serve right away.

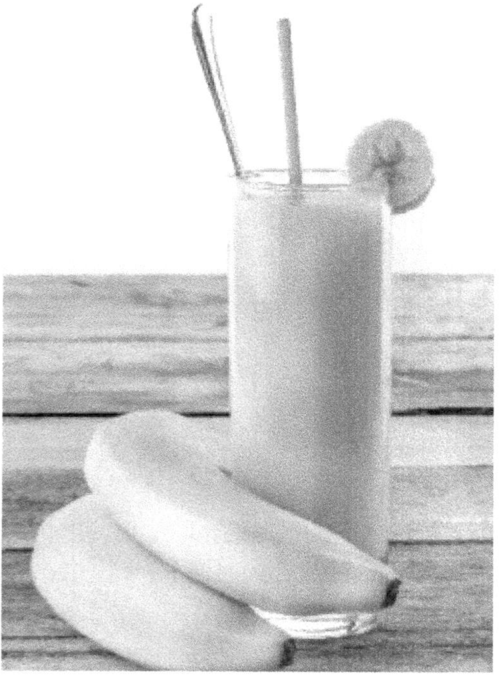

3. Strawberry Banana Protein SmOOTHIE

Active Time: 10 minutes
Total Time: 10 minutes

Ingredients:

- 1 cup of hulled strawberries, fresh
- Four ice cubes
- 1/2 medium bananas
- 1/2 cups of diced mango, fresh
- 1/2 cups of nonfat yogurt, sugar-free

Instructions

1. In a blender, combine strawberries, banana, mango, yogurt, and ice cubes.
2. Puree till completely smooth.

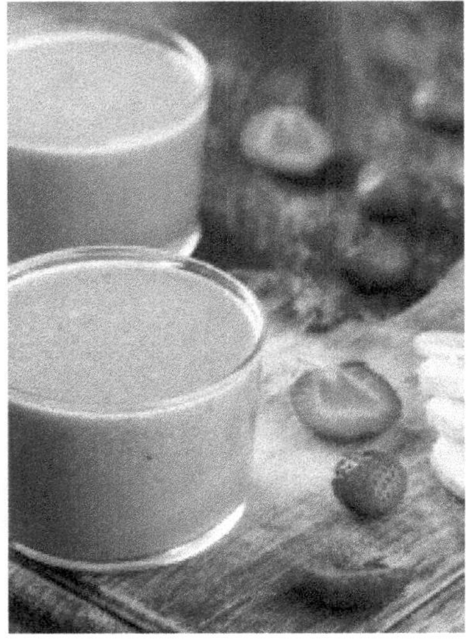

4. Carrot Juice recipe

PREP TIME10 mins
TOTAL TIME10 mins

Ingredients

- 2 ounch carrots
- 1 ounch ice cubes
- Two bananas
- 2 ounces apples

INSTRUCTIONS

1. Thoroughly clean everything with clean water.
2. 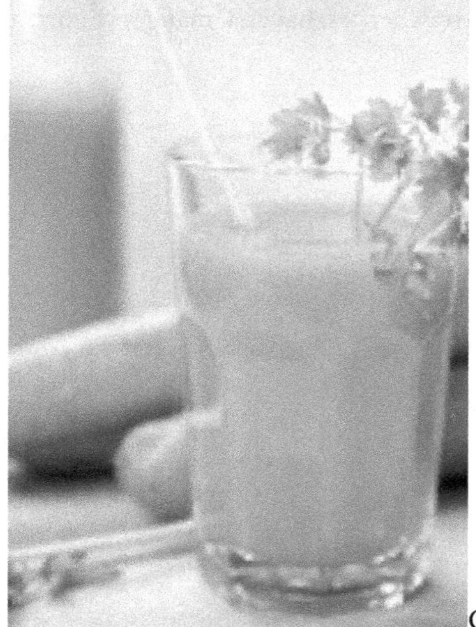Cut apple into bits after peeling it.
3. Peel carrots and cut into quarters vertically.
4. Juice all ingredients in a great juicer.
5. Stir to thoroughly combine juices.

6. Divide juice into tiny amounts and serve with ice cubes.

5. Tropical Fruit Whip recipe

PREP TIME 2 mins
COOK TIME 1 min
TOTAL TIME 3 mins

Ingredients

- 30 g banana protein powder
- ½ cups of ice
- 1 ½ cups of Frozen pineapple
- ½ cups of cottage cheese.

Instructions

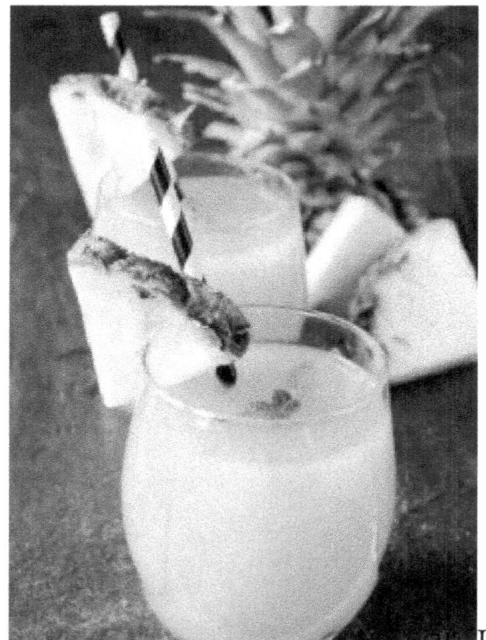

1. In a food processor or blender, combine all ingredients.
2. Blend for 1 min, or until all ingredients are light and pureed.
3. Serve your guests.

6. Mango Yoghurt Recipe

Preparation Time 5 mins
Cook Time 5 mins
Total Time 10 mins

Ingredients

- Mangoes 2 small-sized chopped
- Saffron strands 3-4
- Greek Yoghurt 2 cups, sugar fat-free
- Skim Milk 2 tbsp

Instructions

1. In a mixing bowl, whisk together yogurt till smooth.

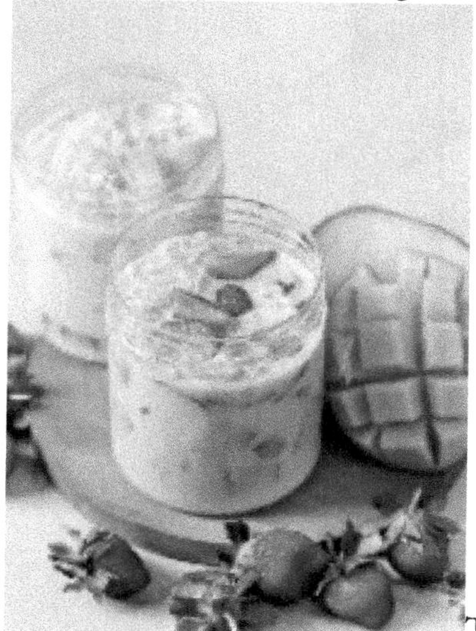

2. Toss diced mango chunks into the yogurt dish and stir thoroughly.
3. Place yogurt and mango mixture in blender and puree till smooth. Toss in the, and.
4. Blend till the purée is smooth.
5. Gently shake the blender jar before pouring it into an airtight glass.

7. Strawberry SmOOTHIE BOWL

Prep 4 min

Ingredients

- 1/2 cups of greek yogurt
- Two strawberries, Frozen
- Two scoops of Whey protein powder.
- 3 tbsp skim milk, unsweetened

Instructions

1. In blender, place strawberries, almond milk, protein powder.
2. Mix strawberry mixture in yogurt.

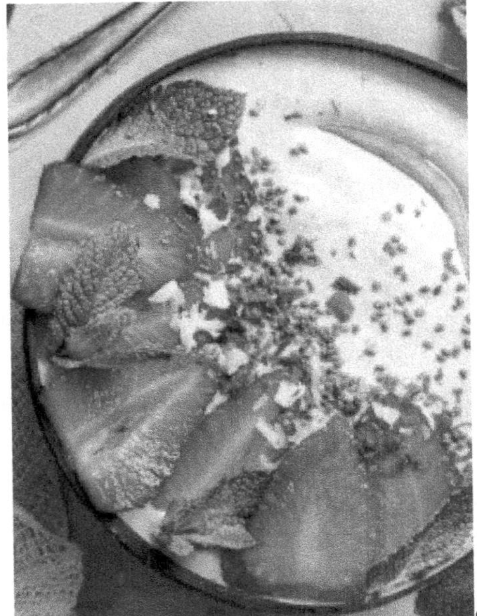

3. Serve

8. Berry Protein Shake HOMEMADE

Total Time
10min

Ingredients

- 3/4 cups of mixed blueberries, raspberries, strawberries
- 1/2 cup of low-fat Greek yogurt.
- ½ cups of a fresh banana
- One scoop of protein whey powder

Instructions

1. Blend all ingredients in the food processor highly.
2. Mix ice cubes and put them in a blender.
3. Serve.

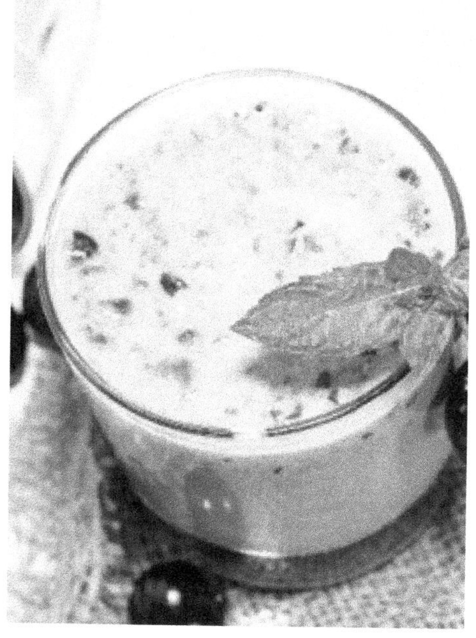

9. SWEET COTTAGE CHEESE FRUIT BOWL

Prep time: 10 mins
Total time: 20 mins

INGREDIENTS

- 1 cup of cottage cheese
- ½ cups of blueberries
- ½ cups of strawberries sliced
- ¼ cups of skim milk sliced

INSTRUCTIONS

1. Mix in 1 cup of the cottage, 1/2 cup of blueberries, 1/2 cup of sliced strawberries, 1/4 cup of milk.
2. Serve.

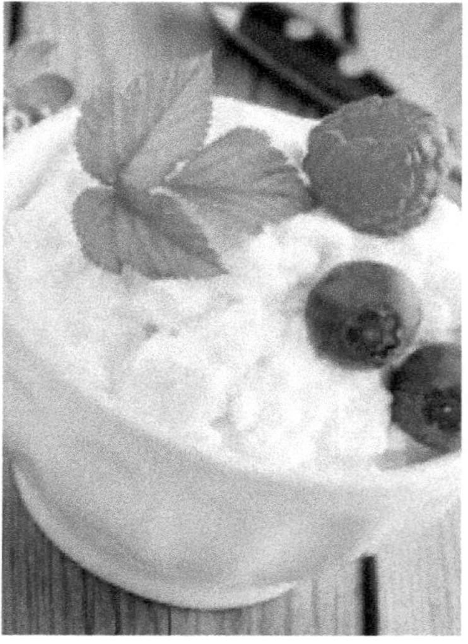

10.Apple Oatmeal recipe

Prep:5 mins
Cook:5 mins
Total:10 mins

Ingredients

- 1 cup of water
- ¼ cups of apple juice
- One apple, cored and chopped
- ⅔ cup of rolled oats
- 1 cup of skim milk

Directions

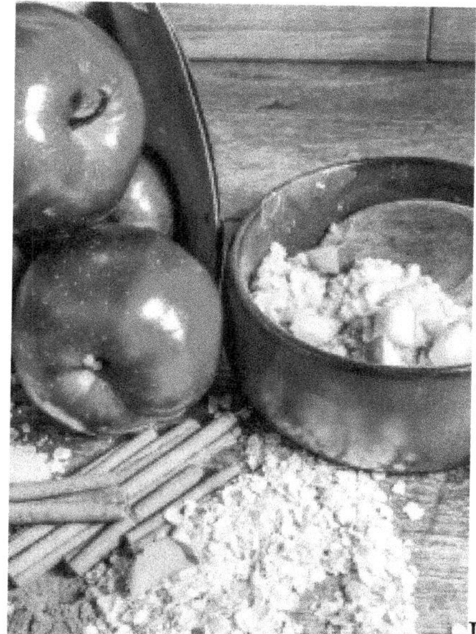

1. In a saucepan, combine apples, apple juice, and high-boiled water.
2. Bring to boil over high heat; ad rolled oats. Bring to boil, then lower to low heat setting.
3. Pour milk over dishes and spoon into serving dishes.

4. Serve

11.Cottage Cheese & Fruits

Prep Time 5 mins
Cook Time 0 mins

Ingredients

- 2 cups of whole strawberries
- 2 cups of cottage cheese

Instructions

- Slice or chop strawberries and serve on 1/2 cup of cottage cheese.
- serve

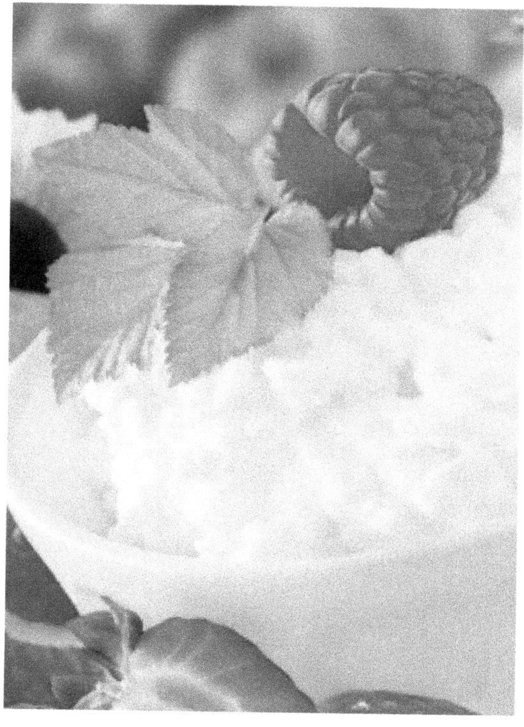

3RD STAGE

SOFT AND MOIST FOODS

You'll start this phase of your diet about two weeks after surgery. Each meal should be roughly the size of 12 cups or 4 ounces, and it should be simple to eat these meals with a fork. You should stop eating as soon as you feel full, regardless of whether this amount has been consumed.

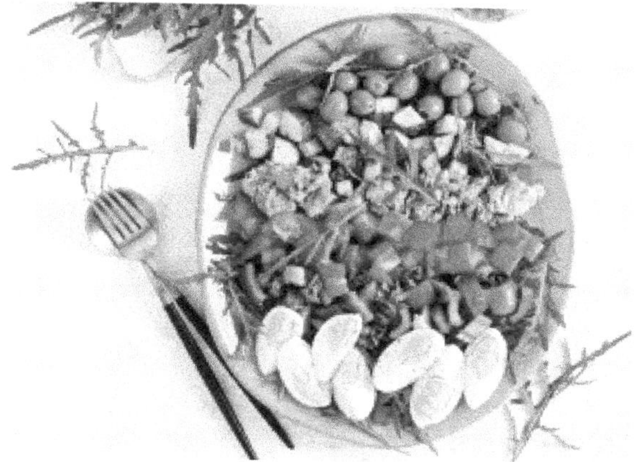

1. CHICKEN ZOODLE SOUP

prep time: 15 mins
cook time: 15 mins
total time: 30 mins

INGREDIENTS:

- 1 tbsp divided olive oil,
- 1 pound zucchini, spiralized
- One sprig rosemary
- 1 pound boneless, skinless chicken breasts, cut into 1-inch chunks
- salt
- Three peeled and diced carrots
- 1/4 tsp dried rosemary
- 4 cups of chicken stock
- water

DIRECTIONS:

1. In a stockpot, heat 1 tbsp of olive oil over medium heat. Taste salt.
2. Add chicken to pot and cook about 2-3 mins till golden; set aside.
3. Place 1 tbsp remaining oil to stock.
4. Mix carrots properly.
5. Cook, occasionally stirring, around 3-4 mins till tender.
6. Remove and rosemary, about 1 minute, before fragrant.
7. Bring to boil in chicken stock and 2 cups water. Incorporate the Zucchini and chicken, reduce heat and simmer till tender, around 3-5 mins.
8. Add; salt and pepper.
9. Serve,

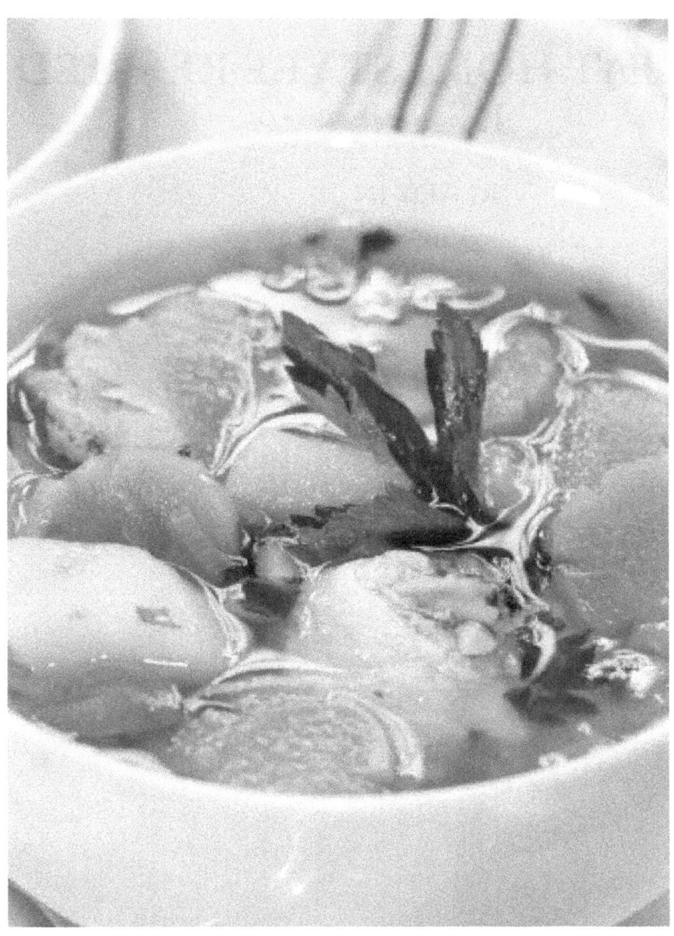

2. LOW-FAT HOMESTYLE REFRIED BEANS

READY IN
15mins

INGREDIENTS

- 1 tsp olive oil fat-free
- Two cans rinsed and drained black beans
- 1/2 cup of water
- 4 tsp lime juice
- 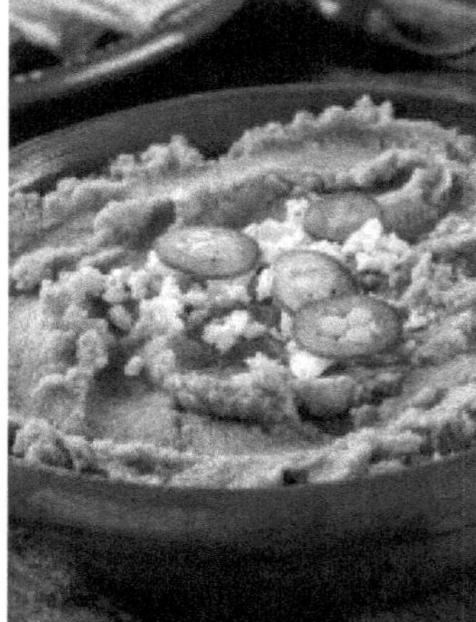1/2 tbsp salt

DIRECTIONS

1. Add bean, salt to the pan
2. Add water, cook, and extract till heated and absorbed by water. It takes just a few mins.
3. Remove and serve

3. Basic Bone Broth homemade

Prep Time 5 mins
Cook Time 8 hrs
Total Time 8 hrs

Ingredients

- 3 pounds bones (chicken)
- 1 tbsp olive oil fat-free
- salt
- 12 cups of water

Instructions

1. Heat stove to 400 F and place on sheet with parchment paper.
2. 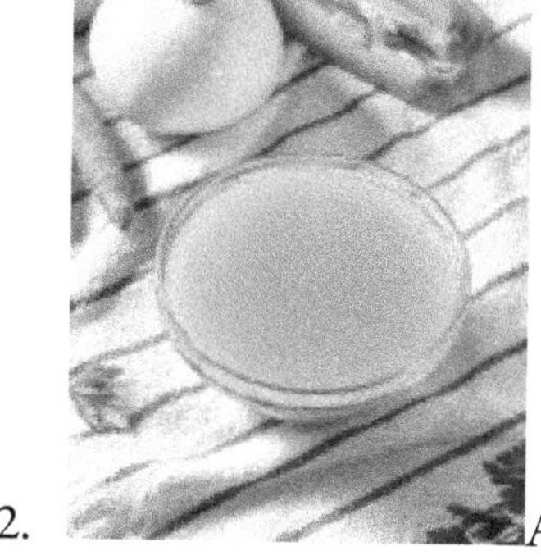Arrange bones and drizzle on a baking sheet with olive oil. Roast 30 mins, or slightly orange. Roast. Switch halfway to facilitate cooking even.
3. Move the bones to a heavy stockpot with pair of tongs. Mix water together.
4. Bring the pot to boil over medium to high heat and turn the heat to low immediately. Simmer, exposed, for a minimum of 8 hours and 16 hours. Skim any foam that appears on the broth's surface.
5. Strain the broth, and season it with fine sea salt. Serve

4. cottage Protein Shake

Prep Time
10 mins

Ingredients

- 1 cup of coconut milk
- 1 cup of ice
- One scoop Whey Protein
- 1½ tsp. cottage cheese

Instructions

1. Set milk, ice, whey protein ladder, and chocolate chips, and blender extract; cover. Mix until it's smooth.
2. serve

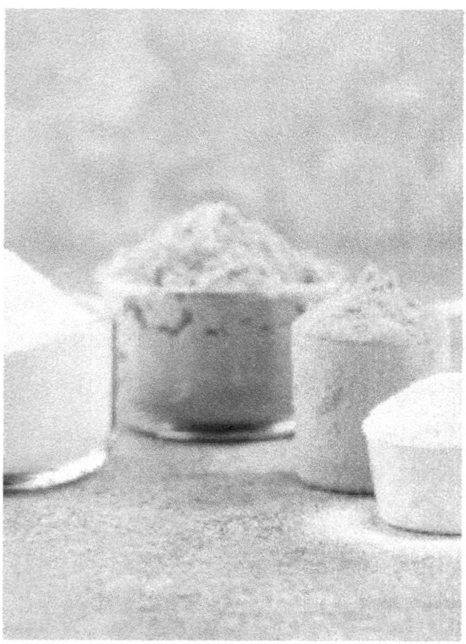

5. black bean soup

Cook time
35 mins

Ingredients

- 1 tbsp olive Oil fat-free
- One can of black beans
- carrot

Instructions

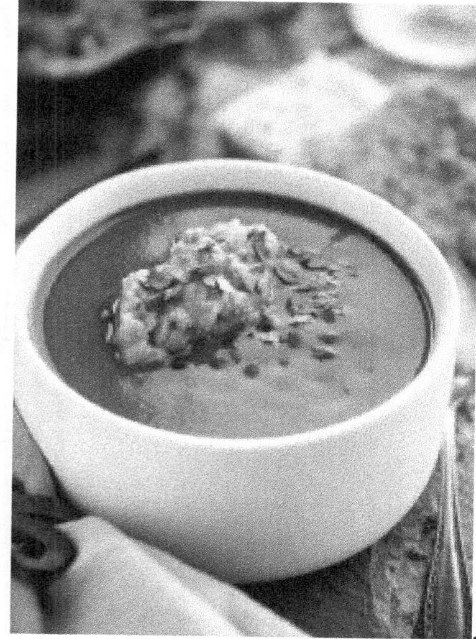

.heat pot with olive oil
.Add carrot and beans.
Cook for 25 mins.
Need cups of beans and blending them.
finally, mix it in a pot and serve

6. Chicken Meatballs recipe

Prep Time:5 mins
Cook Time:20 mins

Ingredients

- 1/2 pounds of Ground Chicken
- 1/4 cups of mozzarella cheese, Shredded
- 1/4 cups of cottage Cheese Shredded

Instructions

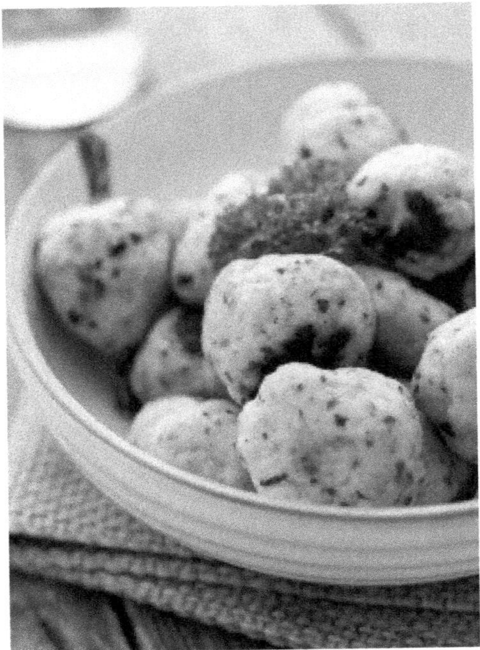

1. Heat oven to 350 degrees Fahrenheit.
2. Combine all ingredients in a medium mixing dish.
3. Form tiny meatballs with about 1 tbsp of the meat mixture
4. Arrange meatballs in the baking tray.
5. Bake meatballs for 15-20 mins, covered.

7. Garlic Pureed Salmon

Prep time 12 mins
Cook time 20 mins

Ingredients

- Four lunch salmon, canned
- Salt
- 1/8 tsp powder, garlic
- Olive oil, fat-free

Instructions

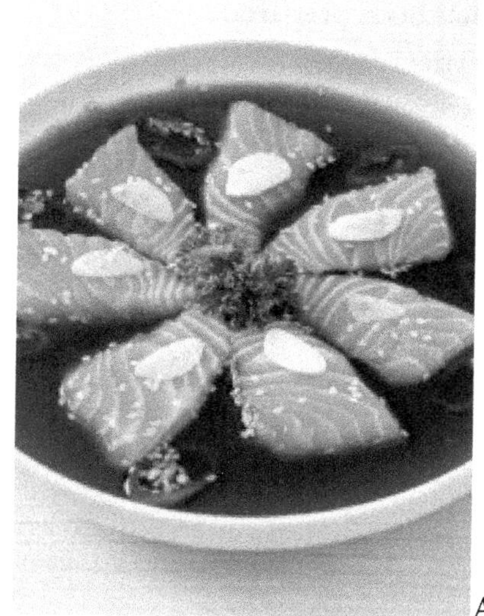

1. At 360 degrees, cheat the oven
2. A baking pot need to take
3. Mix oil on the pot. Place, salt.
4. Place salmon pitches.
5. till 15 mins cook
6. serve hot

8. BANANA COOKIES oats

Prep Time5 minutes
Cook Time14 minutes
Total Time19 minutes

INGREDIENTS

- Three mashed over-ripe bananas
- cups quick oats

INSTRUCTIONS

1. Combine mashed bananas and quick oats in a large mixing bowl.
2. Place on a baking sheet that has been prepared.
3. Bake for 12 to 14 mins at 350 degrees.

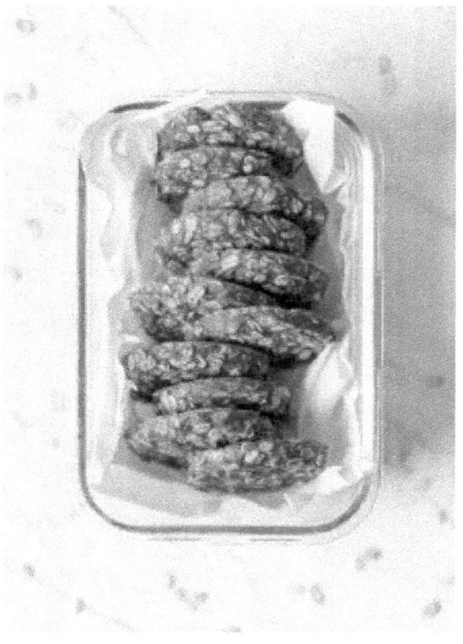

9. Mango Ice Cream recipe

Prep Time
10 minutes
Freezing4 hours

Ingredients

- Two mangoes cut into large chunks
- 1/2 cups of skim milk

Instructions

1. 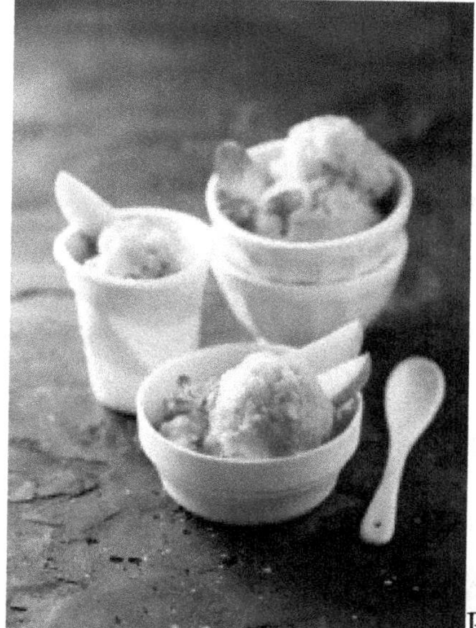Peel and pit mangoes before slicing.
2. Combine mango and sweetened skim milk in the blender.
3. Blend till there are no visible chunks of mango.
4. Transfer mixture to freezer-safe container and freeze for 4 hours.

10. Good Start SmOOTHIE

Prep time 5 mins

Ingredients

- 1/2 cups of the frozen fruit mix, blueberry, banana
- 1 - 100 gram greek yogurt, fat-free, sugar-free.
- 1/2 cups of no sugar added strawberry juice

Directions

1. In a blender, mix and blend ingredients till smooth.
2. Enjoy

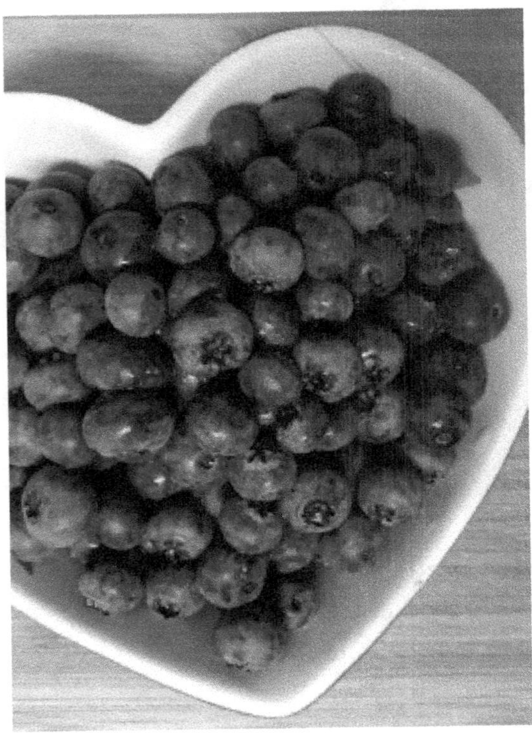

11. Banana Pancakes recipe

Total: 5 min
Active: 5 min

Ingredients

- 1 tsp olive oil, as needed
- Two large eggs
- One ripe medium banana

Directions

1. Heat oil in skillet medium temp.
2. combine eggs and banana till smooth in a blender
3. Cook for 1 minute in a heated skillet with banana mixture.
4. Cook 1 minute on another side.
5. Serve right away

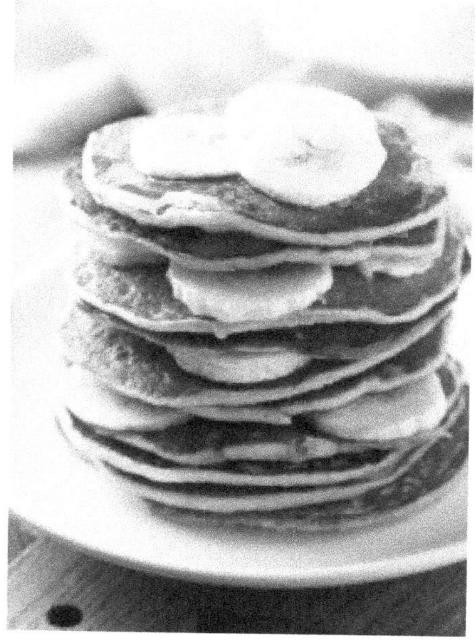

12. Avocado Mango Mash

Prep Time:
15 minutes
Total Time:
15 minutes

Ingredients

- Three avocados, pitted and cubed
- 1/4 tbsp each salt
- One mango pitted and cubed

Instructions

1. 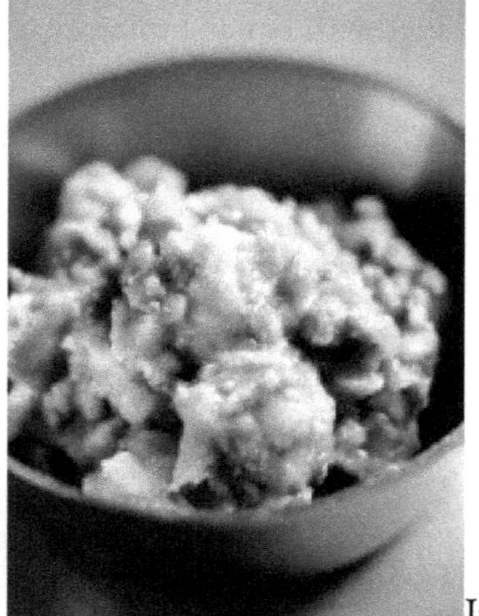In a small bowl, combine avocados, salt. With a fork, mix to desired consistency till fully blended, leaving avocado pieces intact.
2. Combine mango in a mixing bowl. Add a pinch of pepper to mix.
3. Serve.

13. Mango Dairy Lassi

Prep time 5 mins
Total time 5 mins

Ingredients

- ⅓ cups pineapple juice
- 1 cup of chopped frozen mango or mango + banana combo
- ⅓ cups of unsweetened low-fat greek yogurt

Instructions

1. In a blender, mix and blend ingredients till smooth.
2. Serve.

14. BEST GREEN SMOOTHIE RECIPE

Prep Time: 2 minutes
Cook Time: 3 minutes
Total Time: 5 minutes

Ingredients

- 1 cup of fresh spinach
- One banana
- Two strawberries
- 1 cup of water
- 1/2 cups of frozen pineapple
- 1/2 cups of frozen mango

INSTRUCTIONS

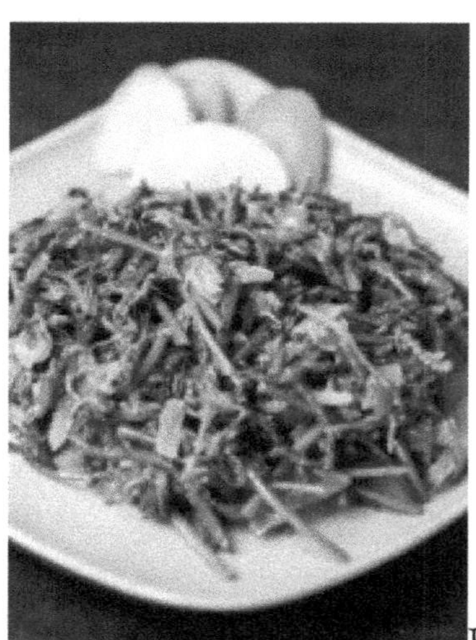

1. Blend spinach with water in a food blender. Blend all together till there are no more lumps.
2. In a blender, combine pineapple, mango berries, and banana.
3. Mix all together till it's smooth and creamy.
4. Serve.

15. Tilapia and Mango Salsa

Ingredients

- 1 Mango
- 4 Tilapia filets canned
- salt
- 1/3 tsp bell pepper
- 1 tbsp olive oil
- One cucumber

Instructions

1. Chop the mango and cucumber into small pieces. Toss the chopped ingredients in a bowl.
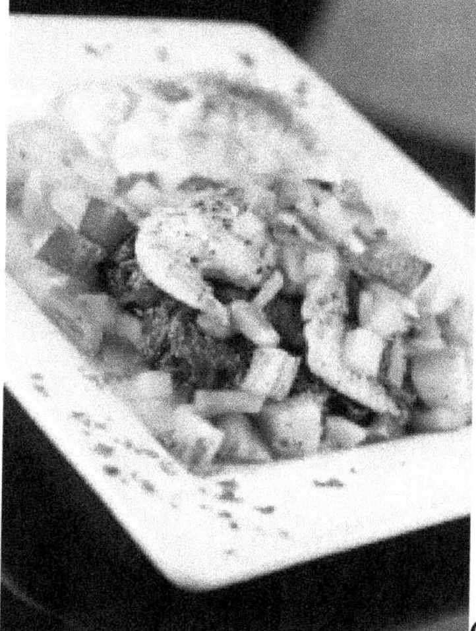
2. Chill for 20-30 mins before serving
3. heat stove to 375 dF.
4. Rinse the fish and pat it dry. Season salt to taste on each fillet. Cook for 8 to 12 minutes in the oven after placing the tilapia on a baking sheet and spraying each fillet with cooking spray.
5. Toss cooked tilapia with mango salsa and serve.

16. MANGO LASSI HOMEMADE

Prep Time 15 minutes
Cook Time 5 minutes
Total Time 20 minutes

Ingredients

- 2 cups of Freshly chopped mango pcs
- Two nos Ice Cubes
- 2 cups of Fresh Chilled curd fat-free
- water

Instructions

1. Peel and cube mangoes into tiny pieces.

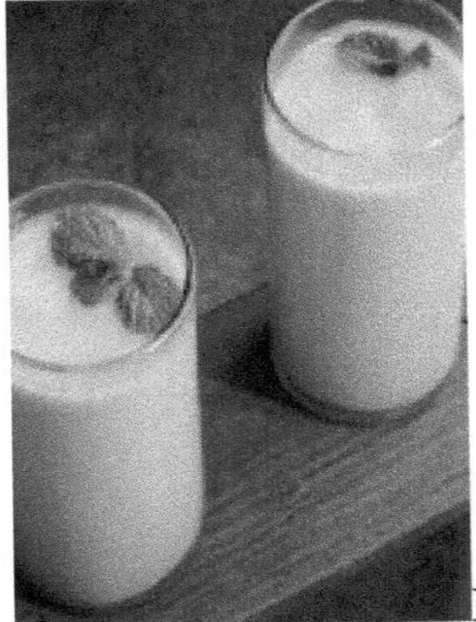

2. In a large blender, combine all of the above ingredients, including mangoes and water, and mix till smooth.
3. Now add cold curd and ice cubes and mix for a few seconds more to get a smooth consistency.
4. To serve, pour the lassi into glasses.

17. Pureed Classic Egg Salad

Prep Time5 mins
Total Time 5 mins

Ingredients

- Two hard-boiled eggs
- Salt
- 1 tbsp reduced-fat mayonnaise
- 1 tbsp yogurt, fat sugar-free

Instructions

1. 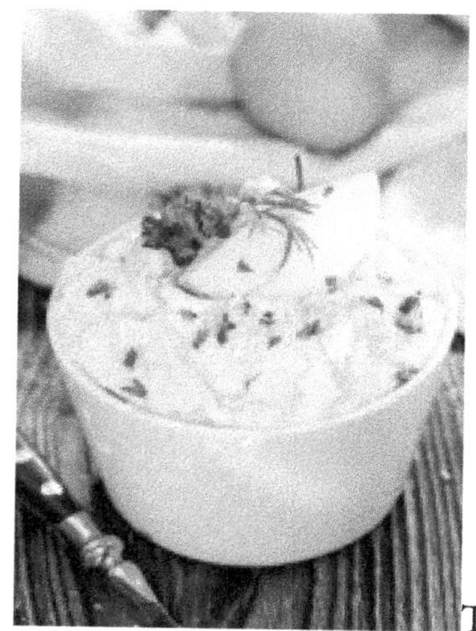Two hard-boiled eggs, sliced
2. Chop eggs till there no big pieces left.
3. Place egg slices in a food processor and pulse till smooth.
4. Toss chopped eggs with mayonnaise, yogurt, and spices.
5. Mix well.

18. Chilled Shrimp Soup

INGREDIENTS

- 2 cups of fat-free skim milk
- salt
- brown sugar
- Stevia
- 1/2 pound cooked shrimp cleaned, peeled

DIRECTIONS

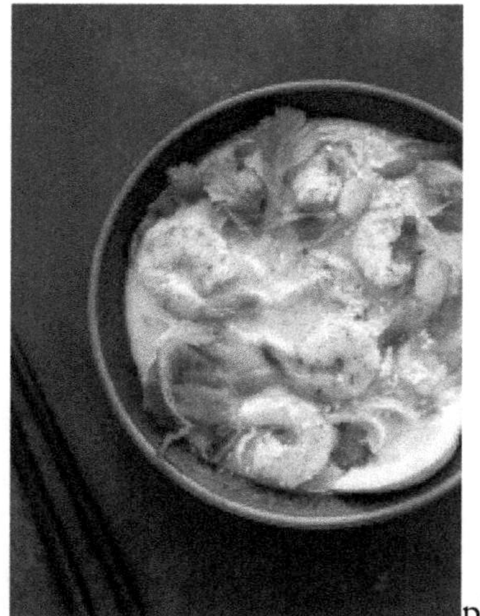

1. place all ingredients in the food processor perfectly
2. puree till smooth
3. mix salt,
4. enjoy!

19. Fresh Fruit Salad

Active:15
minsTotal:
15 Mins

Ingredients

- 2 cups of diced pineapple
- Four ripe kiwis, peeled, halved, and sliced
- 1 pound hulled and sliced strawberries

Directions

1. mix pineapple, strawberries, and kiwi in a large bowl.
2. Serve yogurt dressing.

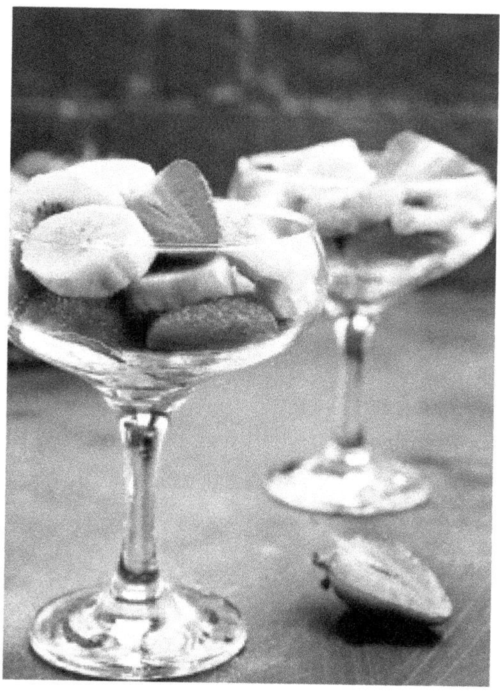

20. High Protein Mousse

Prep Time: 5 minutes
Resting Time: 30 minutes
Total Time: 35 minutes

Ingredients

- One small box Black Cherry
- 1 cup of Water
- Ten ounces Fat-free Greek Yogurt
- One scoops unflavored whey protein powder

Instructions

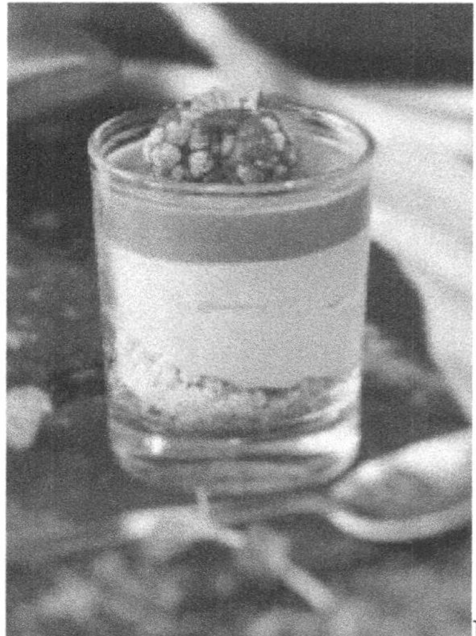

1. Heat water till warm but not boiling.
2. Pour water over cherry in a mixing dish and set it aside while organizing other ingredients.
3. Mix everything in a mixing pan.
4. Pour into four ramekins, put aside to cool.

21. EGG DROP SOUP

prep time: 5 MINUTES
cook time: 5 MINUTES
total time: 10 MINUTES

INGREDIENTS

- 4 cups of low-sodium chicken broth
- 1 tbsp reduced-sodium soy sauce
- Two large eggs, beaten
- 1/4tsp salt
- 2 tbsp water

INSTRUCTIONS

1. 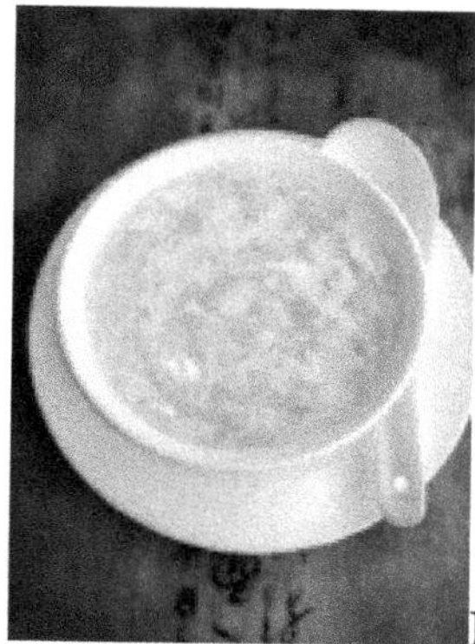Bring chicken stock, soy sauce to boiling in a large saucepan.
2. Add to the boiling soup and stir till it thickens.
3. Lower the heat to a low simmer. Drizzle eggs into the soup slowly while swirling in a circular motion
4. Remove pan from heat and stir in salt.

22. Cheesecake Protein Fruit Dip

PREP TIME
5 mins
TOTAL TIME
5 mins

Ingredients

- Two scoops of whey protein powder
- 8 ounces greek yogurt
- One pkg. sugar-free pudding mix
- 8 ounces skim milk

Directions

1. Whip all ingredients with a mixer till it is light and fluffy.

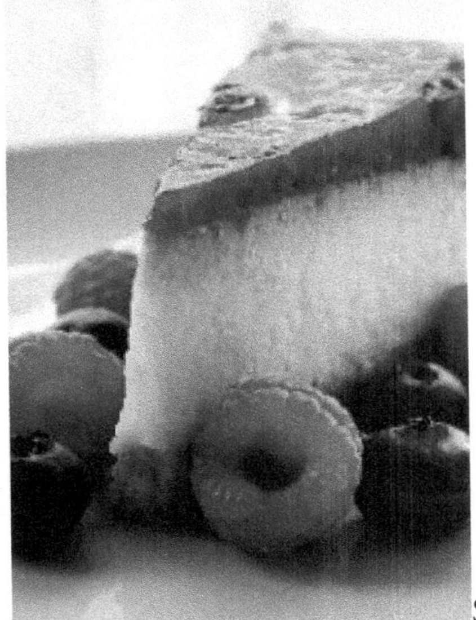

2. Serve.

23. Supreme SmoOTHIE

Prep:5 mins
Total:5 mins

Ingredients

- 2 cups of skim milk
- 2 cups of packed baby kale
- One package of frozen pineapple chunks

Instructions

1. Mix all ingredients in blender perfectly.
2. Blend till smooth.
3. Serve.

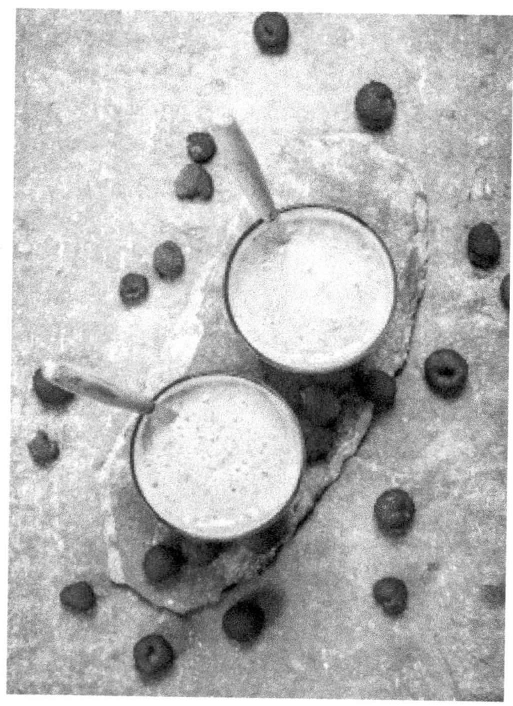

24. Tuna Patties recipe

Prep Time: 15m
Cook Time: 15mins

Ingredients

- Four cans of tuna, packed in water
- Three whole eggs
- 1 cup of grated cottage cheese

Instructions

1. Bake 350 degrees F by mix tuna egg for 25-30 mins, or fry in little olive oil on top of the stove.
2. In a time of 20 mins mix cheese.
3. Serve hot!

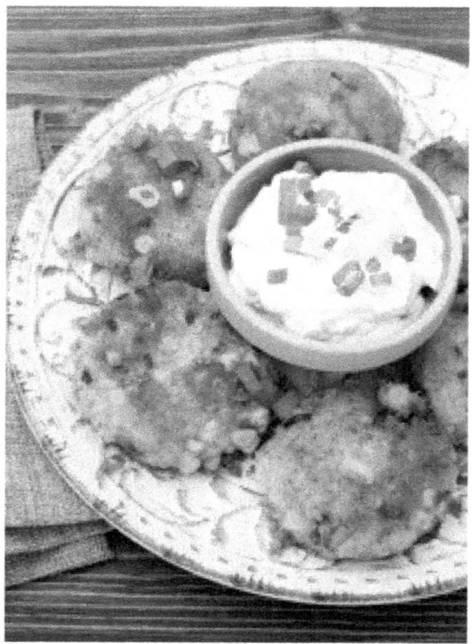

25. EGG SALAD HOMEMADE

Prep Time
15 minutes

INGREDIENTS

- 4 Hard-boiled eggs
- 3 Tbsp mayonnaise Fat-free
- 1 tsp olive oil

DIRECTIONS

1. Peel and chop eggs desired consistency.
2. Mix remaining ingredients.
3. Add eggs and mix well.

26. black BEAN & PLAIN Yogurt

PREP: 5 mins
TOTAL: 5 mins

Ingredients

- 4 cups of plain yogurt fat-free
- Two black beans

Instructions

1. Split beans in half lengthwise, then slice each half-open. Remove little black seeds from the center of beans and toss them into yogurt. To combine, stir thoroughly.
2. Serve

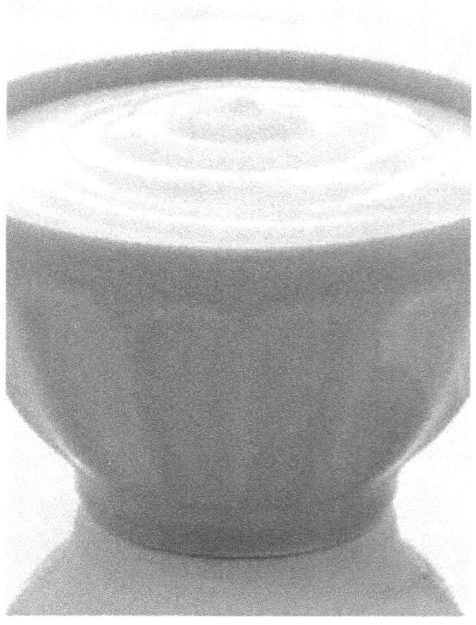

27. The Best Tuna Salad Recipe

Prep Time
5 minutes
Total Time
5 minutes

Ingredients

- Four cans of tuna packed in water drained
- 1 cup of mayonnaise fat-free
- salt

Instructions

1. Combine tuna, mayonnaise in a medium mixing bowl.
2. Salts, mix properly
3. take pleasure in it

28. Mashed Cauliflower HOMEMADE

Prep Time:15 mins
Cook Time:20 mins
Total Time:35 mins

Ingredients

1. One large cut into florets head cauliflower, drained
2. 1/4 cups of cottage cheese
3. Salt

Instructions

1. boil cauliflower and garlic for 10 mins. Separate everything.
2. Combine cauliflower in a blender.
3. Add garlic and pureed cauliflower to the saucepan. Add cottage cheese and taste with salt to suit.

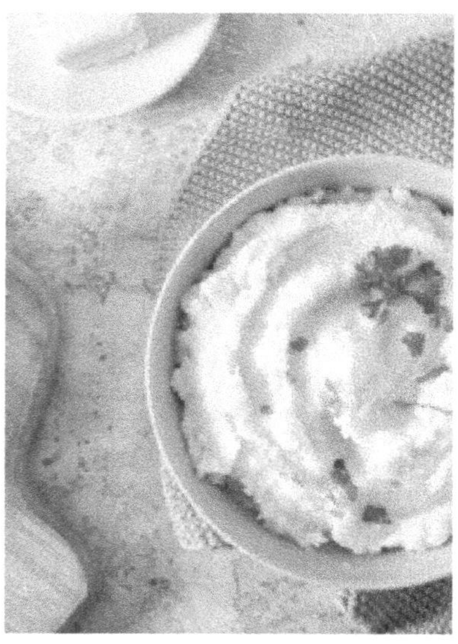

29. Eggs cheese recipe

PREP TIME:2 mins
COOK TIME:2 mins
TOTAL TIME:4 mins

INGREDIENTS

- Four large eggs
- 1 cup of cottage cheese
- Salt
- 1 tsp Olive oil

INSTRUCTIONS

1. Spray oil in a pan on a stove.
2. In a bowl, sprinkle eggs with salt
3. Mix cheese in eggs and
4. Cook for 2 mins
5. Enjoy hot

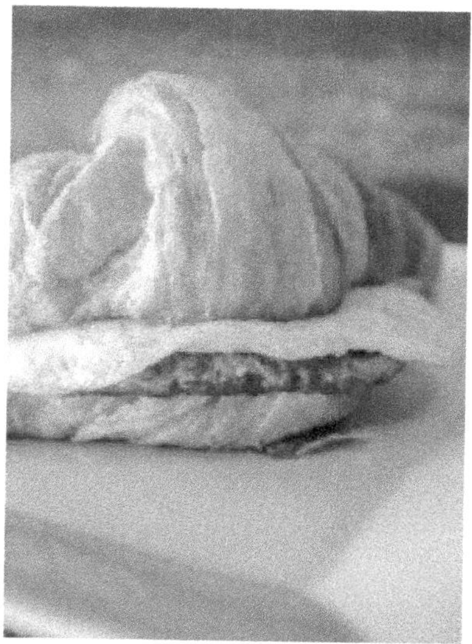

30. Chicken Soup HOMEMADE

PREP TIME 10 minutes
COOK TIME 1 hour
TOTAL TIME 1 hour 10 minutes

Ingredients

- 1 tbsp olive oil
- 8 cups low sodium chicken broth
- 1 ½ cups carrots chopped
- 2 ½ cups cooked chicken
- Salt

Instructions

1. 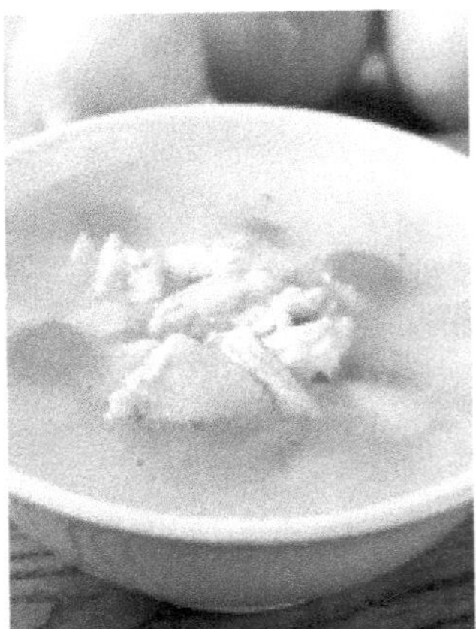Heat olive oil medium heat in a pot. Add carrot, all seasoning.
2. Add chicken with all ingredients.
3. Bring to boil and simmer uncovered for 1 hour or till barley is tender.
4. Give salt.
5. Enjoy now

4th stage

Important stage

AFTER 6 WEEK

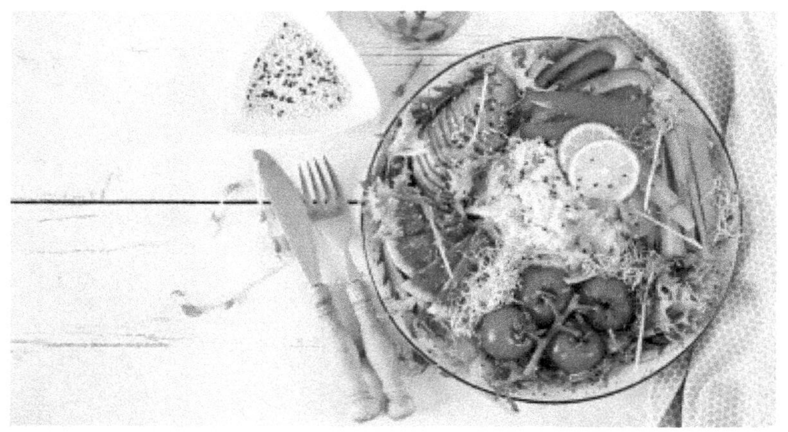

1. Meal Prep Turkey Meatball Zoodles

Prep time:
10 mins
Cook time:
20 mins
Total time:
30 mins

Ingredients

- Four medium Zucchini spiralized
- 2 Cups of Tomato Sauce
- 2 Tbsp Grated cottage Cheese
- 2 Tbsp chopped parsley to garnish

FOR THE MEATBALLS

- 1 1/2 pound Ground Turkey
- 1/4 Cup of mozzarella cheese
- 1 Egg
- 1 Tbsp Italian seasoning
- 1/4 Tsp Chili Flakes
- Salt and ground black pepper

Instructions

1. Heat oven to 400 degrees F and place a sheet of parchment paper in place.
2. Mix all meatballs ingredients in a mixing bowl and stir till mixed. Take mixture spoonfuls and roll between palms to make meatballs.
3. Place meatballs in a prepared baker and cook on sides for 15-18 minutes

4. Divide zoodles into four containers of food storage. Mix sauce, meatballs, cottage, and fresh chopped Persly to garnish.
5. Heat and enjoy.

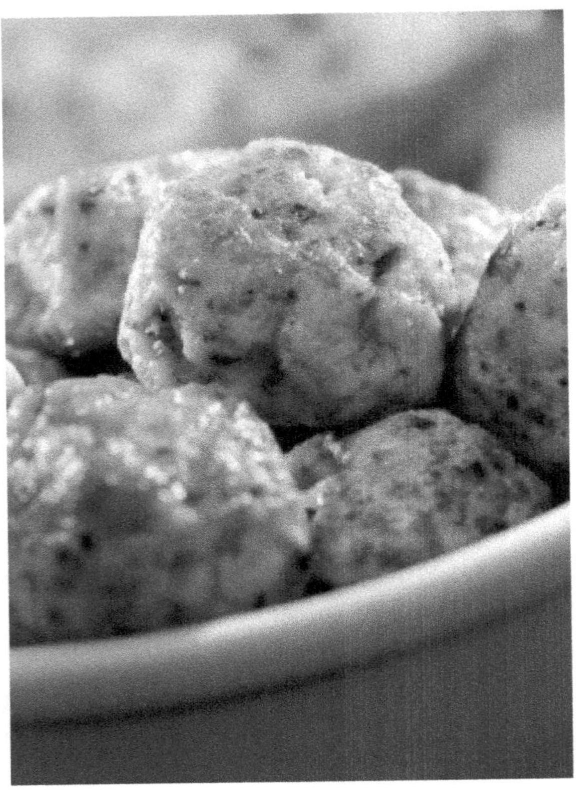

2. Protein Pancakes recipe

Prep Time
5 mins
Cook Time
10 mins
Total Time
15 mins

Ingredients

- 2 Eggs
- 2 Egg white
- Two scoops of Whey Protein powder
- 1 tsp Baking powder
- 6 Tbsp skim milk
- Cooking spray, butter, for grease
- Dark chocolate

Instructions

1. Heat nonstick skillet medium-high heat. Allow melting butter or coconut oil after spraying cooking spray.
2. In a mixing bowl, whisk the eggs, protein powder, and baking powder. Mix almond milk a bit at a time till the mixture is the consistency of pancake batter.
3. Pour batter into skillet using cup measure. When bubbles start to develop on top, they're ready to flip.
4. Toss with butter, sugar-free syrup, and chocolate chips before serve

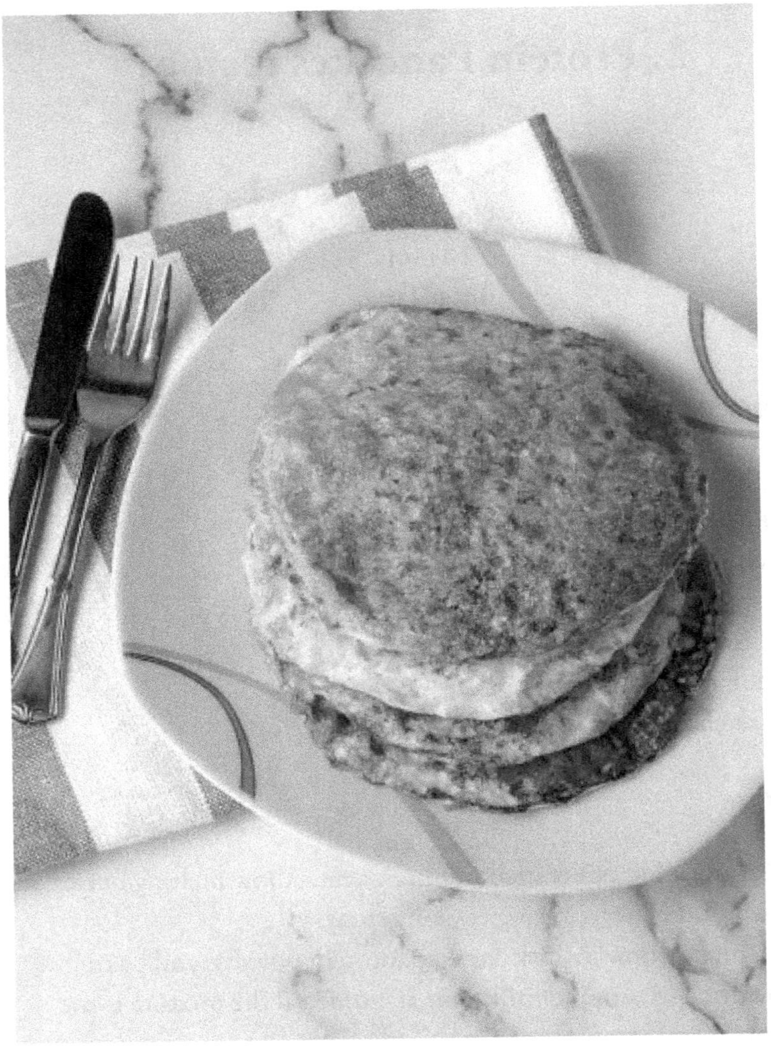

3. Curried Chicken Salad

Prep: 5 min
Cook: 55 min

Ingredients

- Three whole chicken breasts,
- Olive oil
- salt
- 1 tsp black pepper
- 1 1/2 cups of mayonnaise
- 1/4 cups of chutney
- 3 tbsp curry powder

Directions:

1. Heat oven to 350°F.
2. Rub skin of chicken breasts with olive oil and place on a sheet
3. Salt, pepper mix for test
4. Roast for 35 to 40 mins
5. separate bones and skin chicken, divide bite-size pieces.
6. Whisk mayonnaise, chutney, and curry powder with a pinch of salt.
7. Blend till completely smooth.
8. enjoy

4. Shredded Chickens recipe

Cook
time
2 hours

INGREDIENTS

1. 3... 4 pounds boneless skinless chicken thighs
2. Olive oil
3. One diced large onion
4. 1 tbsp black pepper
5. Two minced cloves of garlic
6. 2 tsp paprika
7. 2 tsp salt

INSTRUCTIONS

1. Heat oven to 320 degrees F. Unbox chicken and dry.
2. Heat a drizzle of olive oil in a heavy saucepan over medium heat—Cook for 5 mins with onion and garlic. Stir in paprika. Mix chicken on the plate. Mix salt, black pepper
3. Place saucepan in the oven with a heavy cover on top. Bake for 90 mins, covered. Remove chicken from the oven and place it in a large mixing bowl with a slotted spoon.
4. Serve with lime juice.

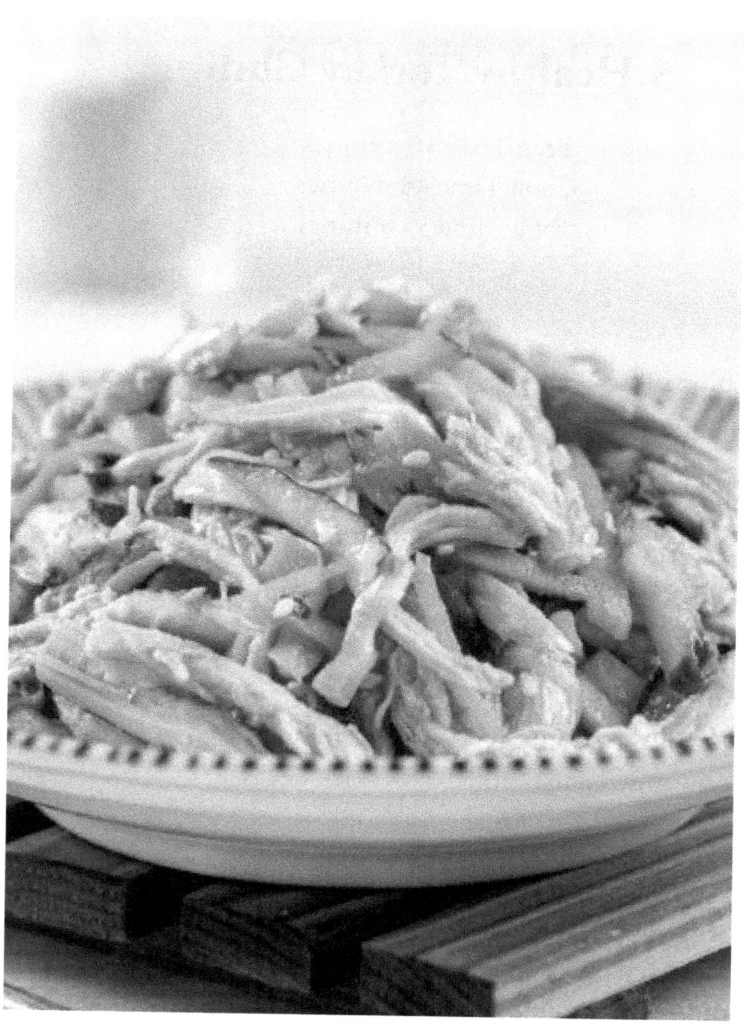

5.Healthy Turkey Chili

Prep Time 10 minutes
Cook Time 45 minutes
Total Time 55 minutes

Ingredients

- 2 tsp olive oil
- One chopped yellow onion
- Three minced garlic cloves
- 1 tsp black pepper
- One can be rinsed and drained sweet corn,
- 1 pound extra lean ground turkey
- 2 tsp ground cumin
- 1 tsp dried oregano
- 1/2 tsp salt
- One can diced tomatoes and crushed tomatoes
- Two cans rinsed and drained dark black beans

Instructions

1. In a large bowl, add oil and heat over medium heat. Stir in the onion, garlic, and red pepper and sprinkle for 5-7 mins.
2. Add turkey on the ground and split meat; cook till not pink anymore. Add cumin, oregano,
3. mix onions, chicken broth, beans. Bring to boil, then reduce heat and cool for 30-45 mins or till chili is thick and flavorful.
4. Garnish with what you want.

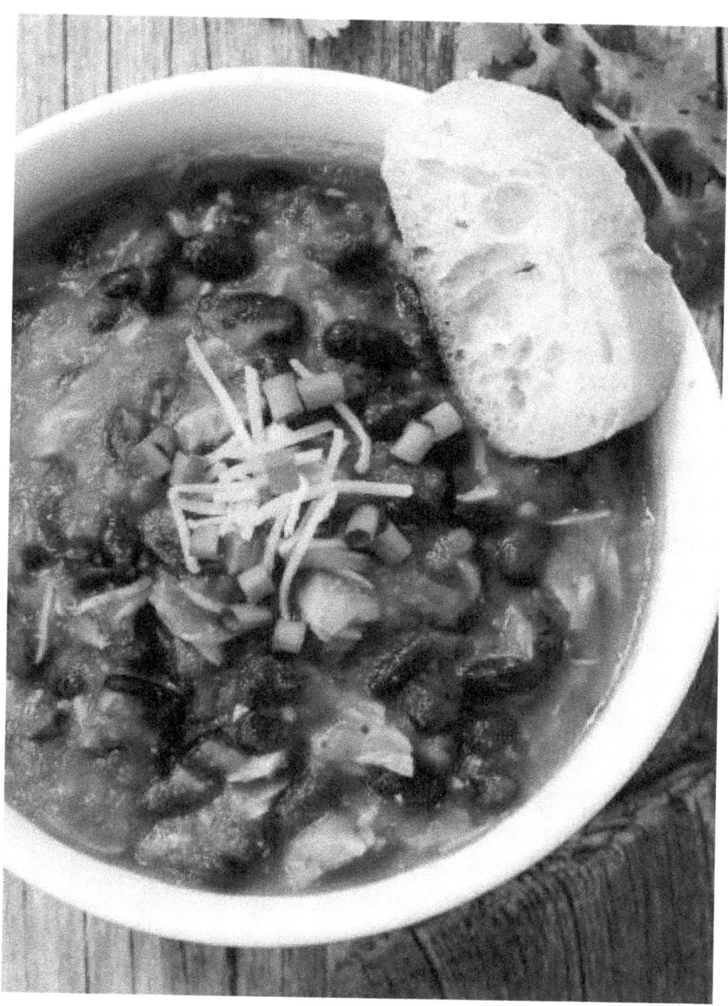

6.Baked Ricotta Florentine

Prep Time
10 mins
Cook Time
15 mins

Ingredients

- olive oil spray,
- 1/2 cups of mozzarella cheese
- 1/4 cups of fresh spinach, chopped fine
- 2 tbsp minced, sun-dried tomatoes
- 8 ounces cottage cheese

Instructions

1. heat the stove to 350 degrees Fahrenheit.
2. Heat an olive oil-sprayed saute pan over medium heat.
3. Olive oil should be used to grease ramekins.
4. In saute pan, cook chopped spinach till wilted.
5. Combine cottage cheese, mozzarella, spinach, and sun-dried tomatoes in a medium mixing bowl.
6. Evenly distribute the mixture among buttered ramekins.
7. Bake for 15-20 mins, or till cheese is slightly browned and melted.

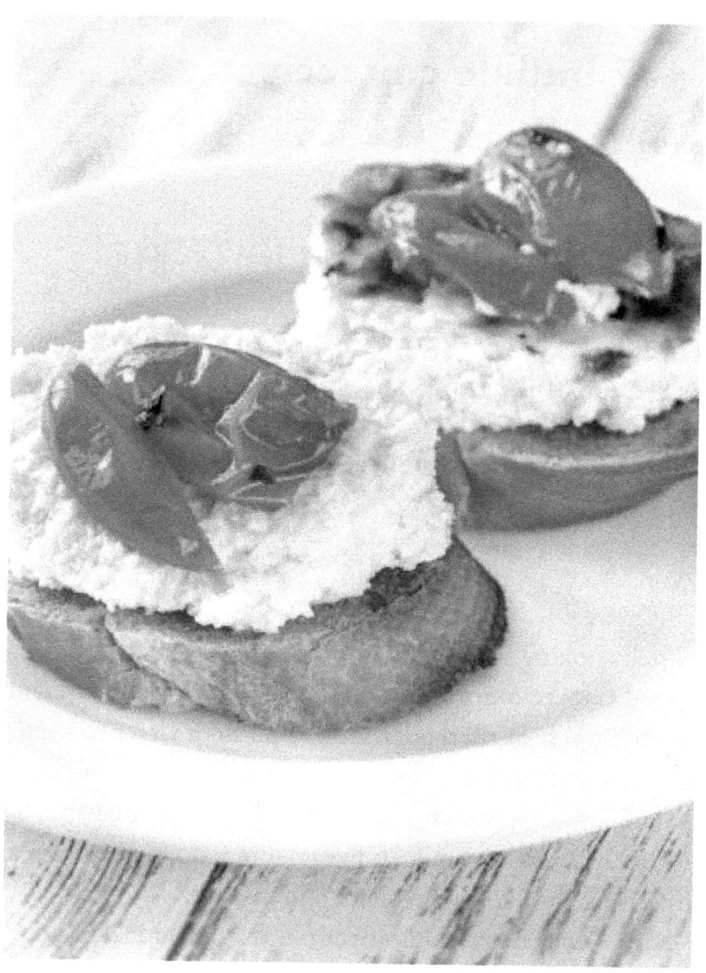

7.buffalo cup recipe

INGREDIENTS

- 1/4 Cups of Chopped Carrot
- 1/4 Cups of Chopped Onion
- 1 Clove Garlic,
- 1 Slice Cheese
- 1/4 Cups of Skim Milk
- 1 Tsp Cornstarch
- 1 Can White Meat Chicken (drained).
- 1 Tbsp Hot Sauce

DIRECTIONS

1. with nonstick cooking spray, Spray frying pan.
2. Add chopped carrots, onion, and smashed garlic clove to pan and cook over medium heat till tender. Add a splash of water to keep onions and carrots from burning.
3. Combine milk and cornstarch in a bowl and stir into the pan mixture. Heat milk, cornstarch, and veggies in a slow, steady stream till the milk thickens. Add spicy sauce and mix well.
4. Remove pan from heat and combine milk, veggies, chicken breast—season with salt, pepper. Divide cheese among servings and spoon chicken mixture into ramekins.
5. Cover with tin foil and bake at 375 degrees for thirty minutes, removing the foil for the final five mins.

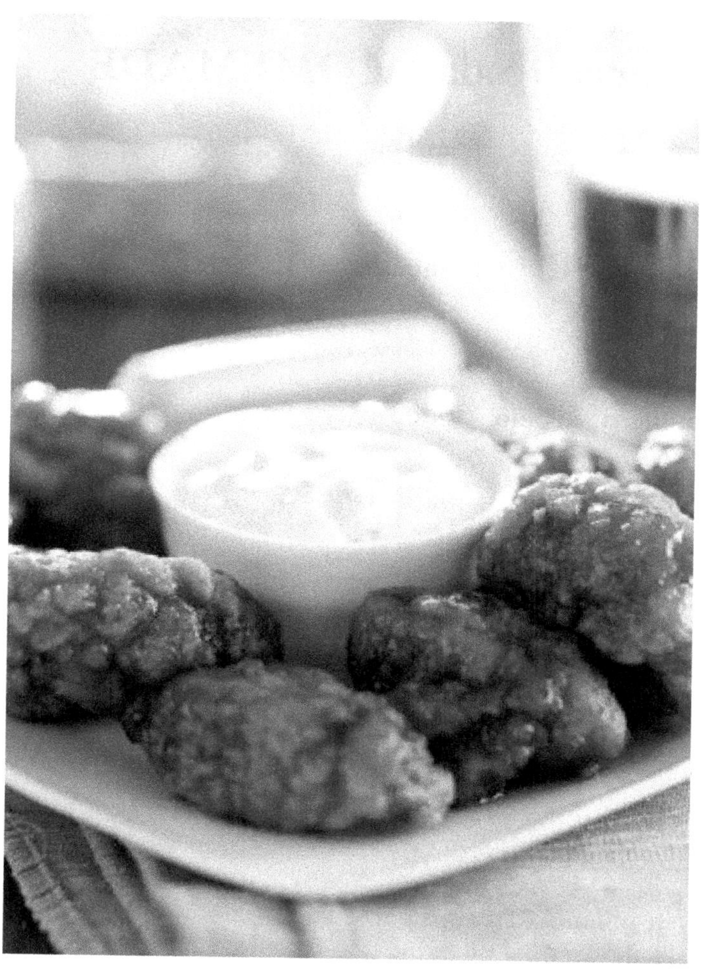

8. Broccoli Salad HOMEMADE

Prep Time
10 minutes
Total Time
12 minutes

Ingredients

- ¼ cup of sliced red onion
- 4/5 cup of broccoli
- Water

Dressing

- ¾ cup of olive oil
- ¼ tsp black pepper
- ½ tbsp lemon juice
- ¼ tsp salt

Instructions

1. Heat oven and mix water in a pot.
2. Mix broccoli and for a 1-minute stay.
3. In another pot, place lemon juice, salt, black pepper, pitched onion.
4. Now mix with broccoli and enjoy

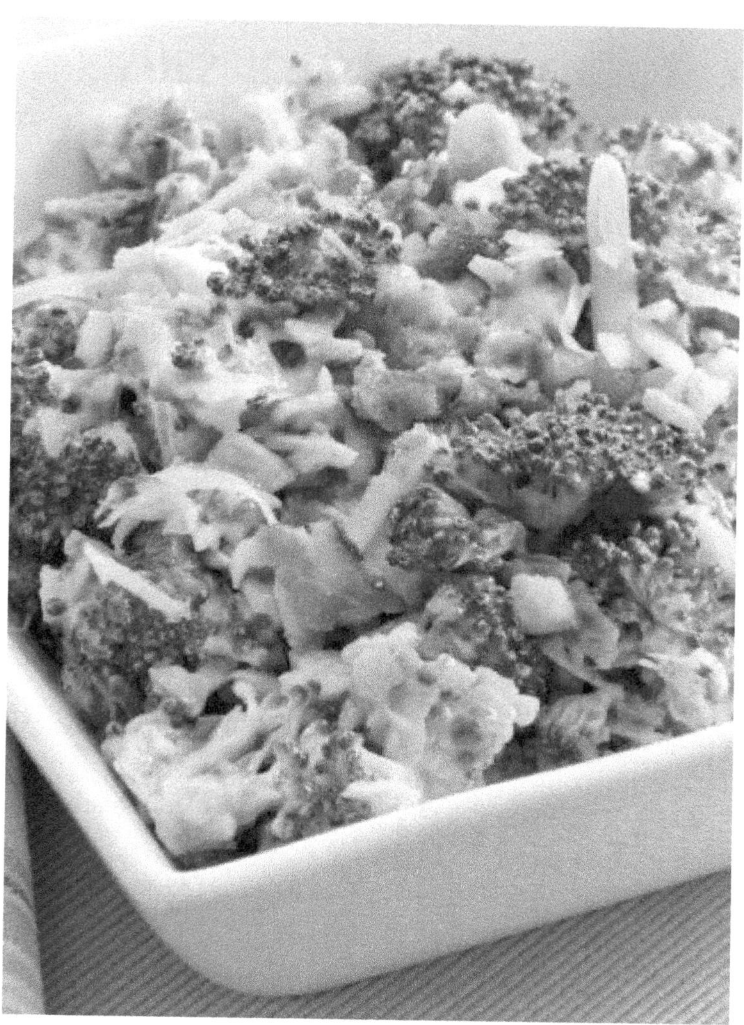

9. Mango Lime and Chilli Salsa

PREP TIME
10 mins
TOTAL TIME
10 mins

ingredients

- One large mango, peeled
- 1 Tsp of red chili, finely chopped
- 1 Medium avocado, chopped
- Black Pepper
- 1 Tbsp. lime juice
- 1 Handful of coriander chopped
- 4 Grape cherry tomatoes, chopped

Instructions

1. Mix all of the ingredients together carefully in a medium-sized mixing bowl.
2. Serve as a side dish with a favorite protein source, such as fish or chicken.

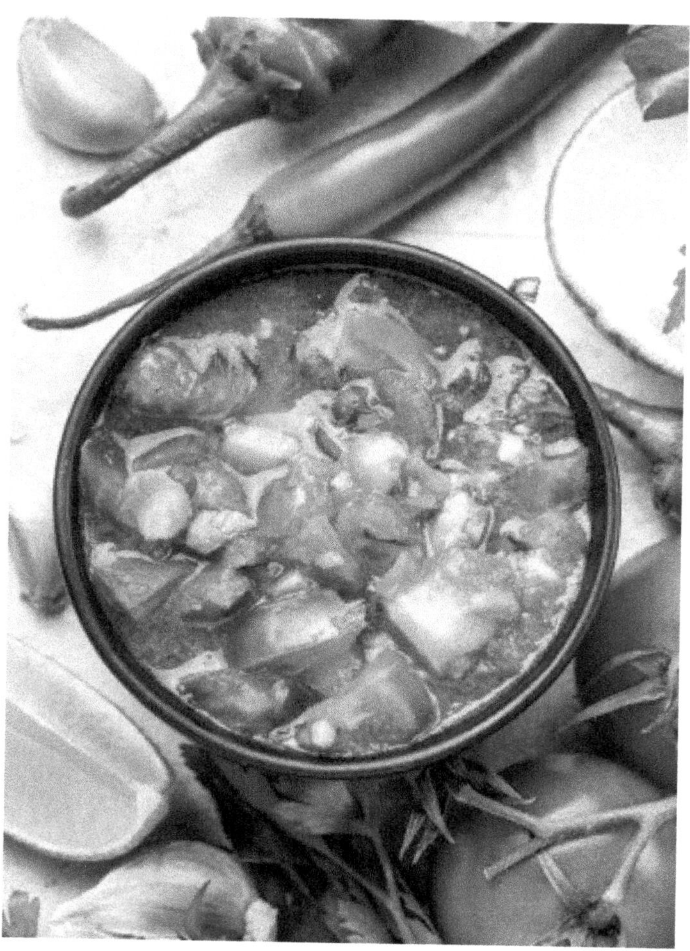

10. Steamed Broccoli recipe

Prep:
10 mins
Cook:
5 mins
Total:
15 mins

Ingredients

- One head of broccoli, cut
- Salt
- 1 tsp black pepper
- Two red bell pepper
- One slice cooked lamb, chopped
- 1 tbsp butter

Directions

1. Place steamer inserts in a saucepan with water till it below the steamer's bottom. Place pot of water to a rolling boil. Mix broccoli, cover, and steam for 3 to 5 mins.
2. In the mixing dish, combine steamed broccoli, lamb, butter, salt, and pepper.

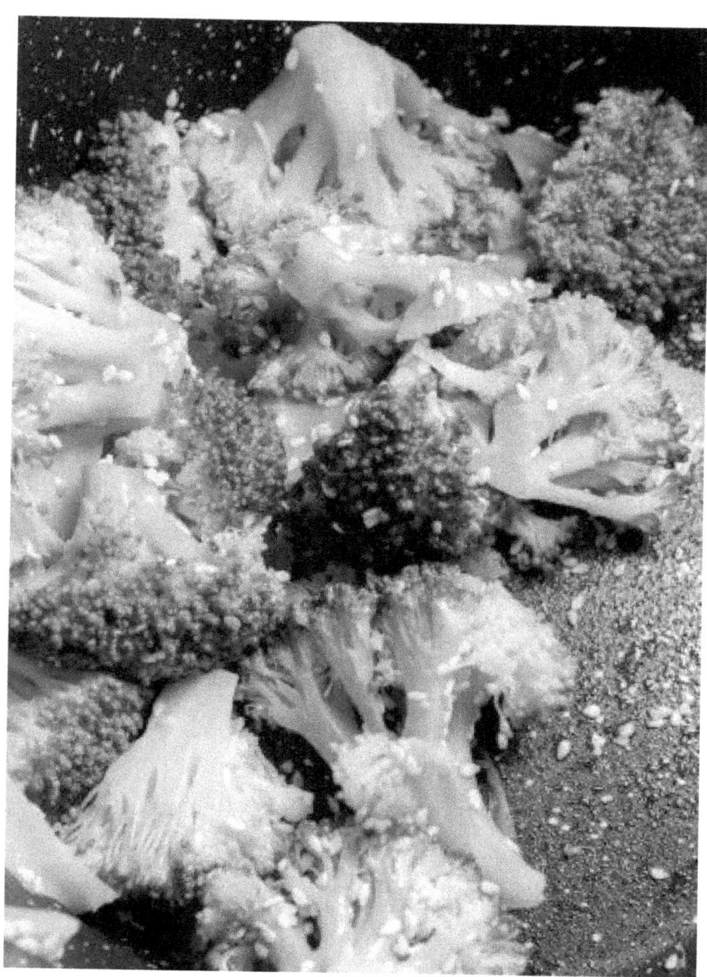

11. Bariatric Peanut Butter Fudge

Prep Time:
5 minutes
Cook Time:
10 minutes
Total Time:
15 minutes

Ingredients

- ¼ cups of Coconut Oil
- 1 tbsp Cocoa Powder
- ¼ cups of whey Protein Powder
- ½ cups of Peanut Butter

Instructions

1. Melt coconut oil in the microwave.
2. Combine melted coconut oil with ingredients in a mixing bowl and whisk till smooth.
3. Pour mixture into silicone muffin tray and place in freezer for 10 minutes to solidify.
4. Have fun!

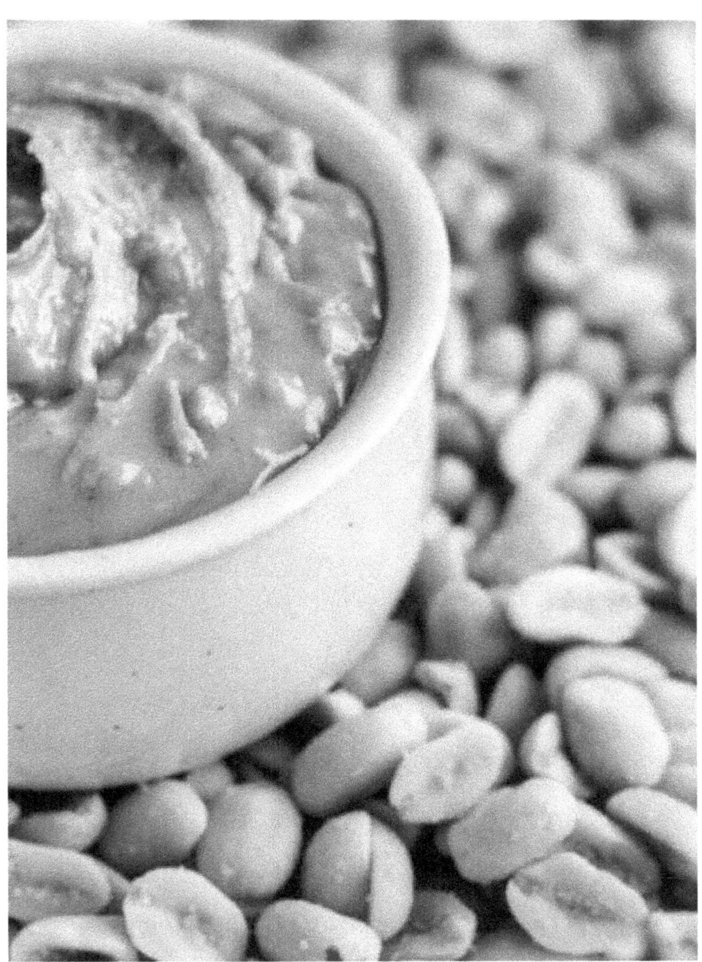

12. BAKED RICOTTA recipe

READY IN: 30mins

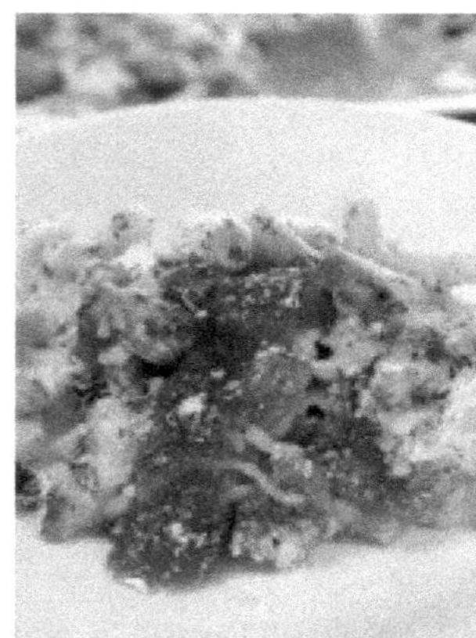

INGREDIENTS

- 8 ounces ricotta cheese
- 1/2 cups of cottage cheese
- One large egg,
- 1 tsp seasoning
- salt
- 1red bell pepper pepper
- 1/2 cups of tomato

DIRECTIONS

1. Mix ricotta, beaten egg, seasonings, and place in an oven-proof dish.
2. Pour sauce on top and top with cottage cheese.
3. Bake it in oven 450 degrees c for 20-25 mins

13. NO-BAKE ENERGY BITES

prep time: 20 MINS
cook time: 0 MINS
total time: 20 MINS

INGREDIENTS

- 1 cup of old-fashioned oats
- 2/3 cups of toasted shredded coconut
- 1 tbsp chia seeds
- 1 tsp honey
- 1/2 cups of creamy peanut butter
- 1/2 cups of dark chocolate chips

INSTRUCTIONS

1. Stir ingredients in mixing bowl till combined.
2. Cover mixing bowl and chill in refrigerator 1-2 hours.
3. Roll mixtures in 1-inch balls.
4. enjoy

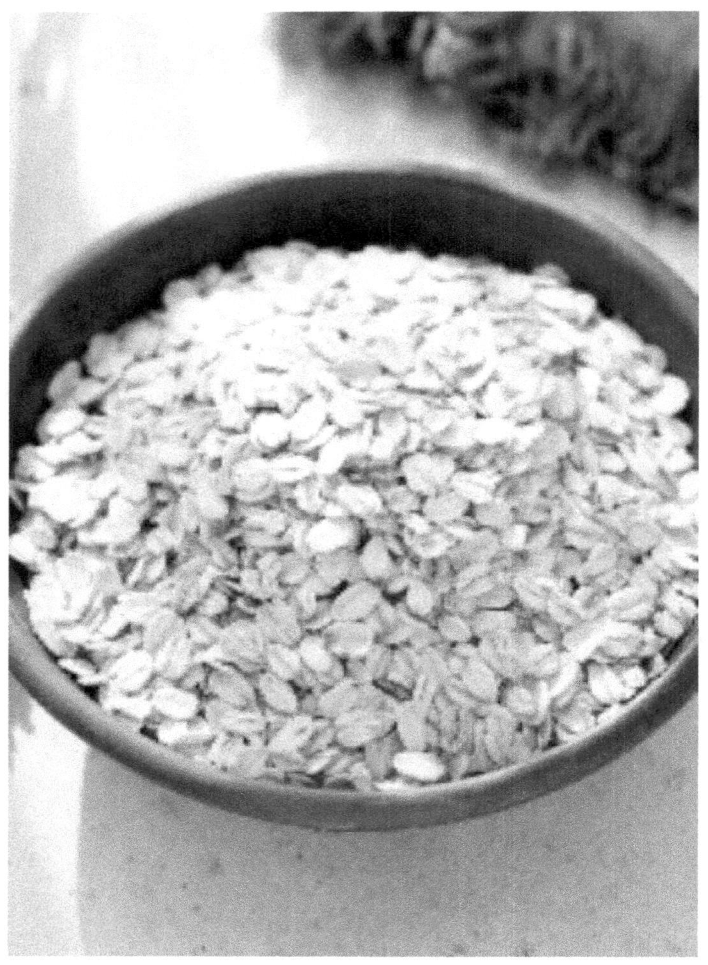

14. Pear and cottage Puree

Prep: 5 Minutes

Ingredients:

- 125g cottage
- 2 tbsp plain, high protein yogurt
- 1/4 tsp cinnamon
- Three pieces tinned pear
- 1/2 tsp honey

Method:

1. Blend all ingredients in the food processor till smooth.
2. To serve, divide into ramekins and top with more cinnamon.

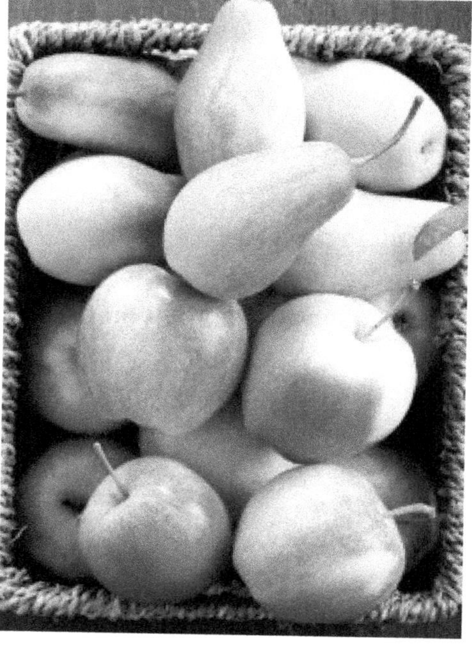

15.Peanut Protein Shake homemade

Prep Time
5 minutes
Blending Time
2 minutes
Total Time
7 minutes

Ingredients

1. 1/2 cup of frozen banana coined
2. 3/4 cups of skim milk
3. 1 tbsp dark cocoa powder
4. 2 tbsp peanut butter
5. 1 scoop of chocolate protein powder
6. ¼ tsp ground cinnamon
7. 8 ice cubes

Instructions

1. Peel banana, then slice it and put it in the fridge.
2. Once the banana is frozen, take 1/2 cup and combine it with milk, cocoa powder, peanut butter, protein powder, ground cinnamon, and ice in a blender.
3. Blend till completely smooth.
4. Serve.

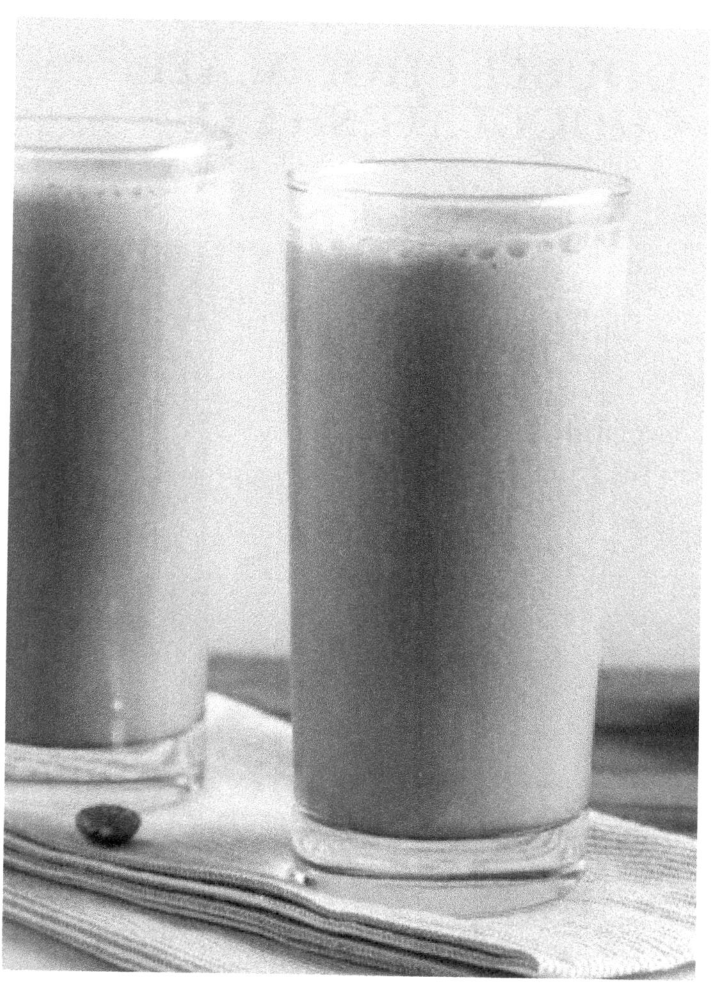

16.DOUBLE CHOCOLATE, CHOCOLATE SHAKE

READY IN: 6mins

INGREDIENTS

- 1 cup of skim milk
- 1 cup of ice
- Four scoops of dark chocolate ice
- Dark chocolate syrup
-

DIRECTIONS

1. Blend milk, chocolate ice, chocolate syrup, and perfectly.
2. 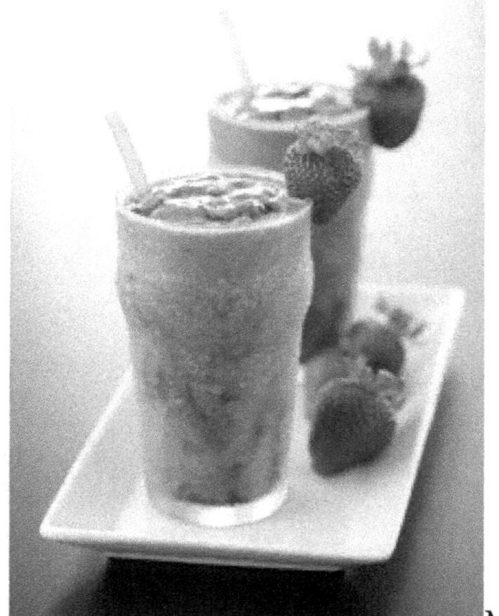Mix ice.
3. Enjoy!

17.Roast side of salmon with chermoula

Prep:15 mins
Cook:15 mins - 20 mins

Ingredients

- 850g side of salmon
- 3 tbsp olive oil
- 1 tsp coriander seeds
- 1 tsp cumin seeds
- ½ small pack mint leaves picked
- ½ small pack coriander
- One lemon, zested
- One fat garlic clove
- ½ tsp chilli

Method

1. Preheat the oven to 200 degrees Fahrenheit/180 degrees Fahrenheit fan/gas 6. Using the baking paper, line the bottom of a roasting tray large enough to hold the salmon—brush 12 tbsp oil all over the skin and season with salt and pepper. Place the salmon in the pan skin-side down and roast for 15-20 minutes, or until it is just cooked through.
2. In a dry frying pan, roast the coriander and cumin seeds. Place all remaining ingredients in a blender and mix until smooth. Blend until smooth, adding enough water to get a drizzling consistency—season with salt and pepper to taste. The chermoula can be made ahead of time and kept refrigerated. Place the salmon on a serving platter and drizzle a little chermoula over it, leaving the rest to serve on the side.

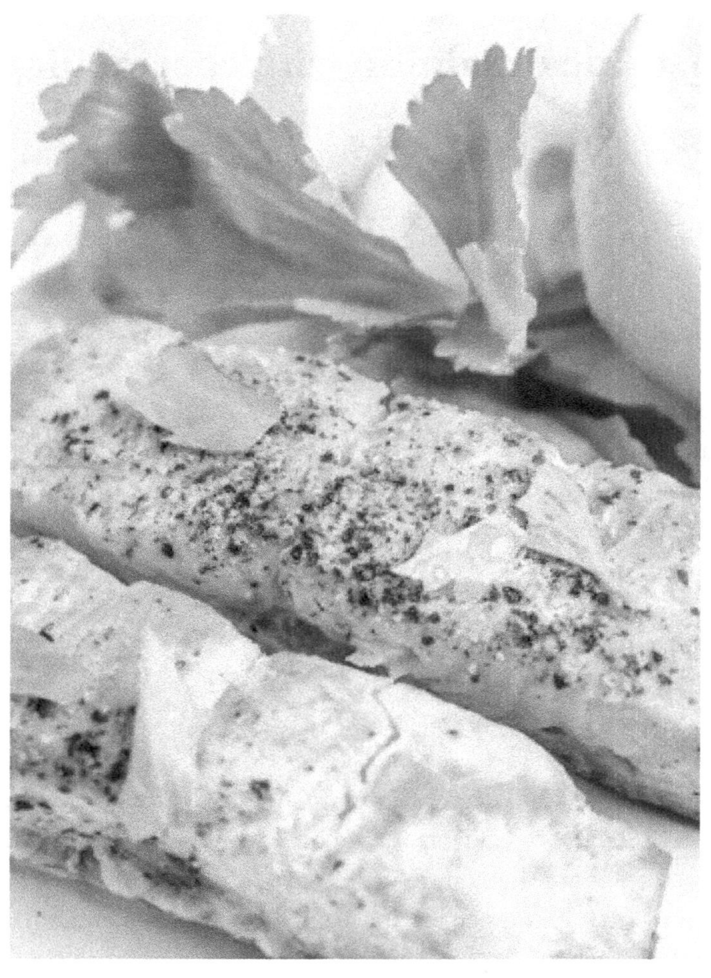

18.Teriyaki salmon with sesame pak choi

Prep:10 mins
Cook:10 mins

Ingredients

- Two skinless salmon fillets
- 1 tbsp sweet chilli sauce
- 1 tsp sesame oil
- 2 tbsp soy sauce
- 2 tsp finely grated ginger
- brown rice or noodles
- For the pak choi
- Two large pak choi
- 2 tsp vegetable oil
- 2 tsp sesame oil
- Three garlic cloves, grated
- 75ml fish or vegetable stock
- 2 tsp toasted sesame seeds

Method

1. Preheat the oven to 200 degrees Celsius/180 degrees Celsius fan/gas six and place two skinless salmon fillets in a shallow baking dish.
2. In a small dish, combine 1 tbsp sweet chilli sauce, 1 tbsp sesame oil, 2 tbsp soy sauce, and 2 tbsp finely grated ginger. Pour over the salmon fillets until fully covered—Preheat oven to 350°F and bake for 10 minutes.
3. Cook the pak choi in the meanwhile. Cut a slit at the base of two big pak choi leaves to separate the leaves.
4. Heat 2 tbsp vegetable oil and 2 tbsp sesame oil in a wok, then add three grated garlic cloves and stir-fry until softened.
5. Fry the pak choi leaves until they begin to wilt. Pour in 75ml fish or vegetable stock, cover firmly, and simmer for 5 minutes - you want

the stems to be soft but still have a bite to them.

6. Serve the pak choi in shallow dishes with the salmon on top, and the liquids spooned over. Serve over brown rice or noodles, if desired, and 2 tbsp toasted sesame seeds.

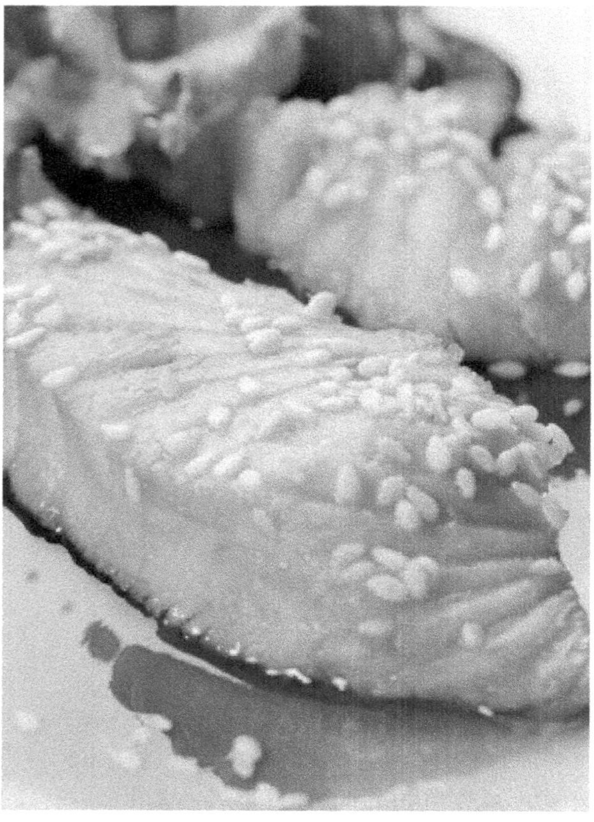

19.Spinach kedgeree with spiced salmon

Prep:15 mins
Cook:45 mins

Ingredients

- 2 tsp olive oil
- One large onion
- a thumb-sized piece of ginger
- ½ tsp cumin seeds
- ½ tsp ground cinnamon
- 6-8 cardamom pods, seeds crushed
- 1½ tsp ground turmeric
- 1½ tsp ground coriander
- One red chilli, deseeded
- One garlic clove, chopped
- One large red pepper
- 70g brown basmati rice
- 375ml vegetable stock

For the salmon

- 3 tbsp fat-free natural yogurt
- 1 tbsp finely chopped mint or coriander
- Two skinless wild salmon fillets
- 1 tbsp toasted almonds, to serve

Method

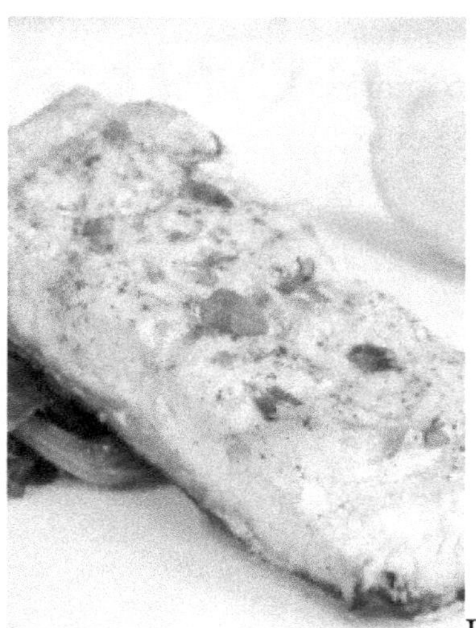

1. In a large frying pan, heat the oil and cook the onion and ginger for 5 minutes, or until tender. 1 tsp turmeric, 1 tsp coriander, cumin, cinnamon, crushed cardamom seeds, cumin, cinnamon, cumin Cook for 30 seconds, or until the mixture is aromatic.
2. Stir in the rice, chilli, garlic, and pepper for a few seconds before pouring in the stock.
3. Cover and cook for 35 minutes, or until the rice is soft and the liquid has evaporated.
4. If the rice is done, but there is still some liquid, remove the lid and continue to cook uncovered to let the liquid drain.
5. Cover and cook for 3 minutes to wilt the spinach.
6. Prepare the fish in the meantime.
7. Preheat the grill to medium and prepare a foil-lined baking pan. Combine the yogurt, mint or coriander, and the remaining turmeric and powdered coriander in a mixing bowl.
8. Spread the yogurt mixture over the salmon, then move to the prepared baking sheet and grill for 8-10 minutes, or until flaking the fish with a fork is easy.
9. To serve, top the kedgeree with salmon fillets or flake the fish into it, then sprinkle the almonds on top.

20.Pesto salmon & bean gratins

Prep:15 mins
Cook:20 mins

Ingredients

- 100g baby spinach
- 3 x 400g cans cannellini beans, drained
- 300g cherry tomatoes, halved
- 2 tbsp olive oil
- 6 tbsp soft cheese
- 150g breadcrumbs
- 40g parmesan, grated
- 3 tbsp pine nuts
- Six salmon fillets
- crusty bread

Method

1. Divide the spinach evenly among six baking dishes (make sure the dishes are safe to use from the freezer to the oven).
2. Drizzle the oil over the beans and tomatoes and serve.
3. As if you were making a salad, toss everything together with your hands.
4. In one dish, combine the soft cheese; in another, combine the breadcrumbs, parmesan, and pine nuts.
5. Season the salmon fillets, place one in each serving dish, and then top with the soft cheese mixture.
6. Sprinkle the cheesy breadcrumbs over the fish and push them in.
7. If you wish to cook right away, preheat the oven to 200°C/180°C fan/gas six and bake the salmon for 20-25 minutes, or until the crumbs are brown.
8. Alternatively, wrap the dishes tightly in plastic wrap and freeze for up to two months; it's a good idea to label the lid with the dish's name

and preparation instructions.

9. Cover and bake for 30-35 minutes at 200C/180C fan/gas six if cooking from frozen.
10. If desired, serve with crusty bread to soak up the juices

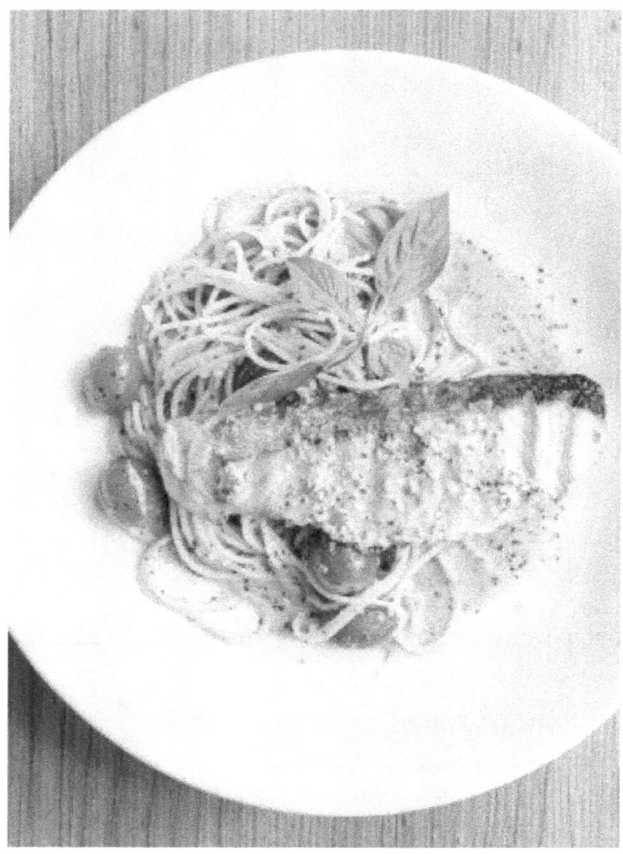

21.One-pan salmon with roast asparagus

Prep:20 mins
Cook:50 mins

Ingredients

- 400g new potato
- 2 tbsp coconut oil
- Eight asparagus spears, trimmed
- Two handfuls of cherry tomatoes
- 1 tbsp apple cider vinegar
- Two salmon fillets, about 140g/5oz each
- handful basil leaves

Method

1. Preheat oven to 220°C/fan 200°C/gas 7 (convection).
2. Place the potatoes in an ovenproof dish with 1 tbsp of olive oil, and roast for 20 minutes, or until they begin to brown. Return the potatoes to the oven for 15 minutes after tossing in the asparagus.
3. Toss in the cherry tomatoes and vinegar, then arrange the salmon on top of the veggies.
4. Return to the oven for a final 10-15 minutes until the salmon is done, drizzling with the remaining oil. Sprinkle the basil leaves on top and serve everything directly from the dish.

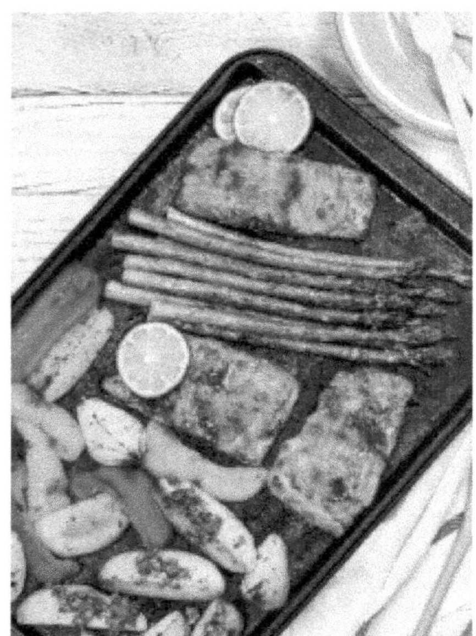

Nutrition

Kcal 483

- Fat 25g
- Saturates 4g
- Carbs 34g
- Sugars 6g
- Fibre 3g
- Protein 33g
- Salt 0.24g

22.Smoked salmon & lemon risotto

Prep:5 mins
Cook:20 mins

Ingredients

- One onion, chopped
- 2 tbsp coconut oil
- 350g brown rice,
- One garlic clove, chopped
- One ½l boiling vegetable stock
- 170g pack smoked salmon
- 85g mascarpone lite
- 3 tbsp flat-leaf parsley, chopped
- grated lemon zest, squeeze of juice
- handful rocket

Method

1. Five minutes in the oil, fry the onion. Cook for 2 minutes, constantly stirring, after adding the rice and garlic.
2. Set the timer for 20 minutes and pour in a third of the stock. Cook, stirring periodically, until the stock has been absorbed, then add half of the remaining liquid and cook, stirring more frequently, until it has been absorbed.
3. Pour in the remainder of the liquid, mix, and cook until everything is done and creamy.

1. Remove the pan from the heat and stir in the diced salmon, cheese, parsley, and lemon zest.
2. Add a pinch of black pepper but no salt because the salmon will be salty enough.
3. Allow 5 minutes for the flavours to meld, then taste and add a splash of lemon juice if desired.

4. Serve with some rocket and the reserved salmon

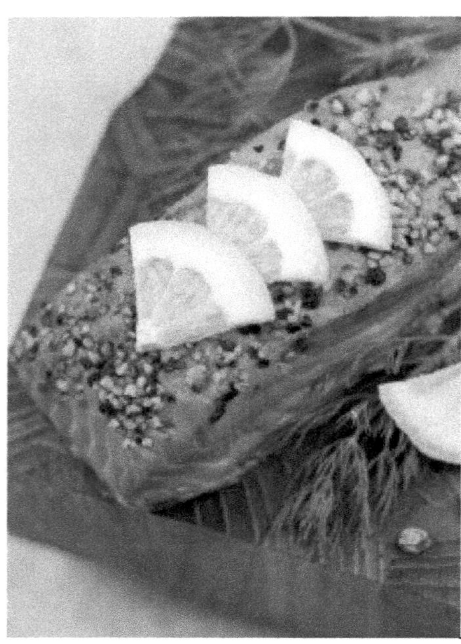

Nutrition:

Kcal 500

Fat 15g

Saturates 5g

Carbs 75g

Sugars 5g

Fibre 4g

Protein 21g

Salt 2.58g

23.Creamy garlic, lemon & spinach salmon

Prep: 5 mins
Cook: 15 mins

Ingredients

- Two sweet potatoes
- 1 tbsp olive oil
- Two salmon fillets, skin removed
- Two garlic cloves, thinly sliced
- 170g baby spinach
- One lemon, zested and ½ juiced, ½ thinly sliced
- 5 tbsp milk

Method

1. heat the oven to 200 degrees Fahrenheit/180 degrees Fahrenheit fan/ gas 6. Microwave the sweet potatoes on high for 5 minutes, or until tender, after piercing them a couple of times (alternatively, bake for 35-40 mins). Maintain a warm temperature until ready to serve.
2. In a frying pan, heat half the oil and gently brown the salmon on both sides - don't worry about it being fully cooked at this stage. Remove the salmon to a dish and clean off the pan before reheating the remaining oil.
3. Cook for 30 seconds without allowing the garlic to burn, then add the spinach, lemon zest and juice, and a pinch of salt and pepper. Cook until the spinach has wilted, stirring in the 2 tbsp milk.
4. Toss the spinach mixture with the lemon slices and salmon fillets in an ovenproof dish. Bake for 5-8 minutes, or until the salmon is fully cooked.
5. Meanwhile, remove the sweet potato flesh from the skins and mash with the remaining milk and a pinch of salt and pepper. Along with the salmon and creamy spinach, serve the sweet potato mash.

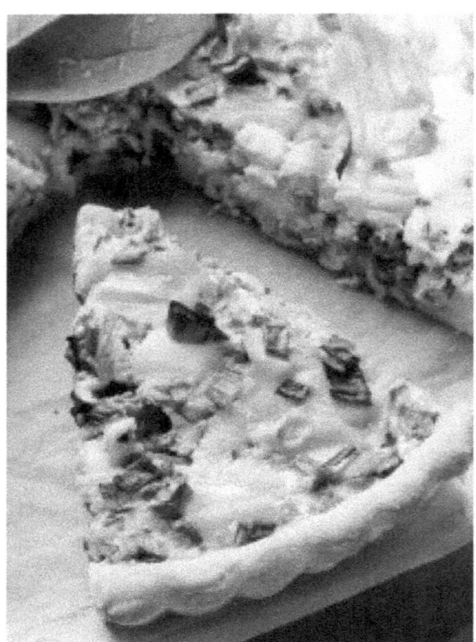

Nutrition

Kcal 721

- fat 44g
- saturates 16g
- carbs 34g
- sugars 19g
- fibre 7g
- protein 43g
- salt 0.5g

24.Fragrant coconut, salmon & prawn traybake

Prep:10 mins
Cook:30 mins

Ingredients

- 1 tbsp sunflower oil
- 5 tbsp red curry paste
- Two garlic cloves, grated
- a thumb-sized piece of ginger, peeled
- 2 x 400ml cans coconut milk
- One red chilli halved
- 1 tbsp fish sauce
- Four thick salmon fillets,
- Four baby pak choi, cut
- 150g mangetout
- 150g raw king prawns
- ½ small bunch of coriander
- 2-3 limes, cut wedges
- cooked jasmine rice

Method

1. preheat oven to 200°C/180°C fan/gas mark 1 6. In a deep frying pan or wok, heat the oil and cook the curry paste, garlic, and ginger for 1 minute.

2. Add the coconut milk and chilli and bring to a low boil. If using, add the fish sauce and lime leaves.

3. Place the salmon, pak choi, in a medium roasting pan with the mixture.

4. Cover and bake for 15 minutes in the oven. Cook for another 10 minutes after adding the prawns.

5. Serve with lime wedges and rice, garnished with coriander.

Nutrition

kcal801
- fat 61g
- saturates 33g
- carbs 13g
- sugar 8g
- high in
- fibre 6g
- protein 46g
- salt2.4g

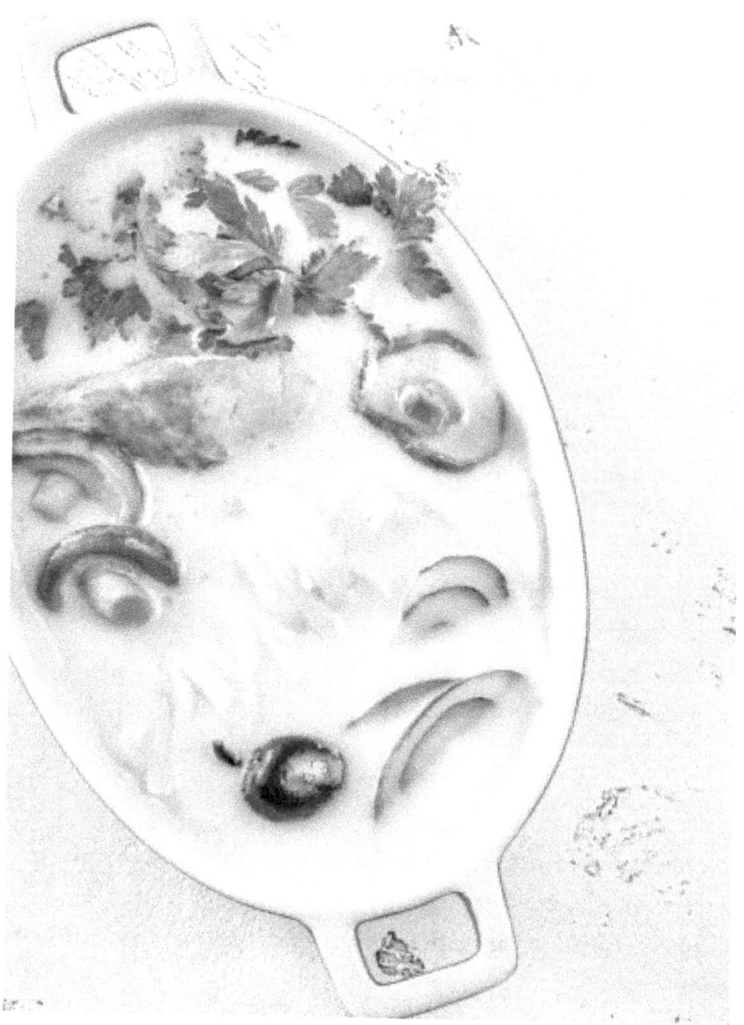

25.Salmon & purple sprouting broccoli grain bowl

Prep:10 mins
Cook:10 mins

Ingredients

- 2½ tbsp coconut oil
- ½ tsp honey
- One lemon, juiced
- 200g broccoli
- 1-2 garlic cloves, sliced
- 250g pouch mixed grains
- handful dill, chopped
- 160g radishes, cut
- 200g cooked salmon, broken

Method

1. 2 tbsp oil, honey, mustard, lemon juice, and spices Bring a pot of water to a boil in a separate pan.
2. Cook for 3-4 minutes, or until the broccoli is cooked but still has a bite, then drain.
3. In a frying pan, heat the remaining oil.
4. Add the garlic and cook for a minute, then add the mixed grain bag and separate the grains with the back of your spoon. Combine the broccoli, mustard dressing, herbs, and radishes in a mixing bowl.
5. Mix everything, season to taste, and then carefully stir in the salmon.

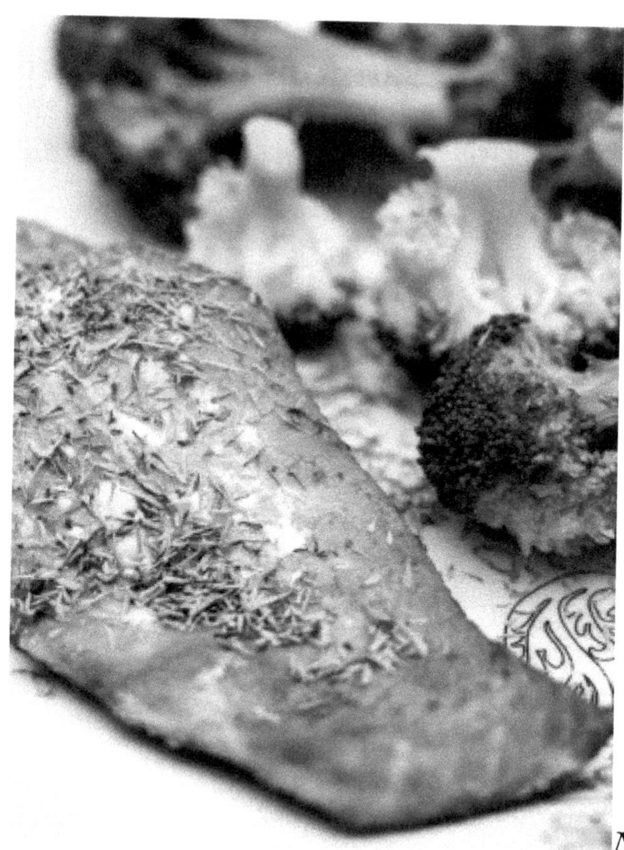

Nutrition

kcal669

fat 39g

saturates 5g

carbs 36g

sugar 6g

fibre 10g

protein 39g

salt0.4g

26.Next level salmon

Prep:
30 mins
Cook:
40 mins

Ingredients

For the cure

- 50g flaky sea salt
- 25g brown sugar
- 2 x 500g skinless, boneless salmon fillets

For the en croûte

- 75g watercress, chopped
- 200g cream cheese
- 2 tbsp fresh dill sprigs, chopped
- One lemon, zested and juiced
- flour for dusting
- Two eggs, yolks only, beaten

For the pickle

- One cucumber, peeled,
- One red onion,
- 100ml apple cider vinegar

Method

1. Combine the salt and sugar in a bowl the day before you wish to construct the en croûte. Scatter half of the salt mix on a tray, then place one of the salmon fillets skinned-side down on top and top with

the remaining salt mix. Sprinkle the remaining salt mixture on top of the second fillet, skinned-side up. Place another tray on top of the first. Refrigerate the tray for up to 48 hours, or at least 12 hours, after weighing it down with a couple of tins.

2. Unwrap the salmon fillets, rinse them in cold water, and pat them dry with kitchen paper. At mixing bowl, combine watercress, cream cheese, dill, lemon zest and juice, smoked salt and a good grinding of pepper. Set aside.
3. Using parchment paper, line a baking pan. Half of the dough should be rolled out on a lightly floured surface to a diameter 2.5cm bigger than the salmon fillet, then draped over the prepared baking pan.
4. Place one of the fillets, skinned-side down, on the crust and cover with the cream cheese mixture, top with the second fillet, skinned-side up. Brush a bit of the beaten yolk along the edge of the crust. The rest of the dough should be rolled out to fit, then draped over the salmon and tucked in at the sides. To seal the edges, trim them and crimp or push with a fork. Brush the en croûte with extra beaten yolk, then chill for 30 minutes before using a spoon to make a scale-like appearance along the top of the dough. Refrigerate for up to 24 hours or at least another 30 minutes.
5. warm oven to 220 degrees Celsius/200 degrees Celsius fan/gas 7. Bake for another 20 minutes before glazing with the remaining yolk. Reduce heat to 180°C/160°C fan/gas four and bake for another 20 minutes, then remove and set aside for 10 minutes.

1. Put the cucumber and onion in a bowl to prepare the pickle. Bring the vinegar and a bit of salt to a boil in a saucepan. Pour the sugar over the vegetables, mix thoroughly, and put aside after it has dissolved. It may be prepared and stored in the refrigerator for up to two days. Serve.

Nutrition

kcal619

fat 43g

saturates 16g
carbs 24g
sugars 5g
fibre 3g
protein 32g
salt2.1g

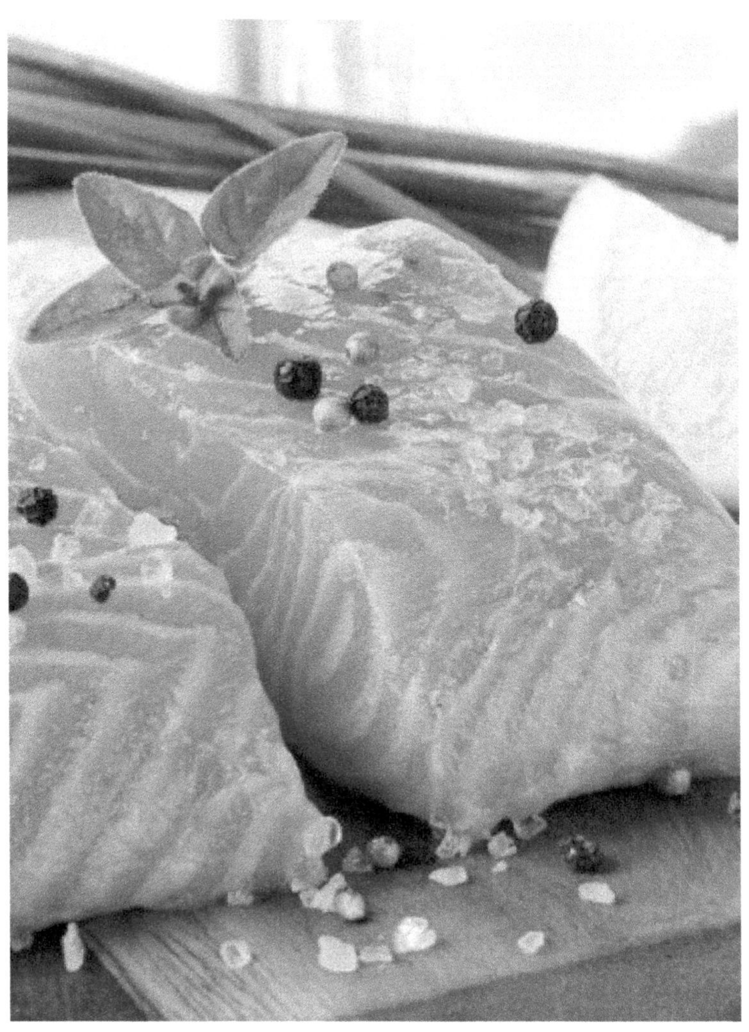

conclusion

| Page

CPSIA information can be obtained
at www.ICGtesting.com
Printed in the USA
LVHW032123201122
733502LV00009B/802

9 798215 735589